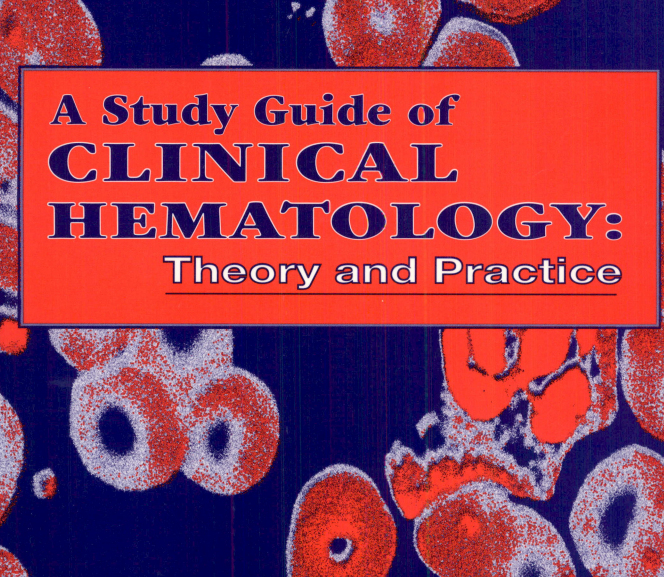

A Study Guide of
CLINICAL HEMATOLOGY:
Theory and Practice

Janice L. Hudson
Robert F. Bunting, Jr.

A Study Guide of Clinical Hematology: Theory and Practice

A Study Guide of Clinical Hematology: Theory and Practice

Janice L. Hudson, MSA, MT(ASCP), SH, DLM
Formerly Assistant Professor of
Medical Technology
Columbus College
Columbus, Georgia

Robert F. Bunting, Jr., MSA, MT(ASCP), CPHQ
Director of Quality and Risk Management
The Medical Center
Columbus, Georgia

Instructor, Graduate Program
Columbus College
Columbus, Georgia

Illustrations by Debra K. Mann, MT(ASCP)

 F. A. Davis Company · Philadelphia

F. A. Davis Company
1915 Arch Street
Philadelphia, PA 19103

Printed in the United States of America

Last digit indicates print number: 10 9 8 7 6 5 4 3 2 1

Acquisitions Editor: Jean-François Vilain
Production Editor: Arofan Gregory
Cover Design By: Donald B. Freggens, Jr.

As new scientific information becomes available through basic and clinical research, recommended treatments and drug therapies undergo changes. The authors and publisher have done everything possible to make this book accurate, up to date, and in accord with accepted standards at the time of publication. The authors, editors, and publisher are not responsible for errors or omissions or for consequences from application of the book, and make no warranty, expressed or implied, in regard to the contents of the book. Any practice described in this book should be applied by the reader in accordance with professional standards of care used in regard to the unique circumstances that may apply in each situation. The reader is advised always to check product information (package inserts) for changes and new information regarding dose and contraindications before administering any drug. Caution is especially urged when using new or infrequently ordered drugs.

Library of Congress Cataloging-in-Publication Data

Hudson, Janice L.
  A study guide of clinical hematology : theory and practice /
Janice L. Hudson, Robert F. Bunting, Jr. ; illustrations by Debra K. Mann.
      p.   cm.
  Includes bibliographical references and index.
  ISBN 0-8036-4604-6
    1. Blood—Diseases—Outlines, syllabi, etc.   2. Blood—Diseases—
Examinations, questions, etc.   I. Bunting, Robert F., 1960–
II. Title.
    [DNLM: 1. Blood Cells—outlines.   2. Blood Cells—programmed
instruction.   3. Hematologic Diseases—outlines.   4. Hematologic
Diseases—programmed instruction.   5. Hemostasis—outlines.
6. Hemostasis—programmed instruction.   WH 18 H885s 1994]
RB145.H76   1994
616.1′5—dc20
DNLM/DLC   93-41166
for Library of Congress   CIP

To Mike and Jim, who made as many sacrifices as the authors.

J.L.H.

To Carmen, Jason, Amanda, and my parents, whose continuous support made the completion of this project possible.

R.F.B., Jr.

Preface

——— ❧ ———

The knowledge explosion in all fields of science has made life increasingly difficult for students. Designed at the request of laboratory science students, this study guide contains an extensive overview of clinical hematology referenced to the following textbooks:

Harmening DM: *Clinical Hematology and Fundamentals of Hemostasis*, ed. 2. Philadelphia, FA Davis Company, 1992.

Lotspeich-Steininger CA, Stiene-Martin EA, Koepke JA (eds): *Clinical Hematology: Principles, Procedures, Correlations*. Philadelphia, JB Lippincott Company, 1992.

McKenzie SB: *Textbook of Hematology*. Philadelphia, Lea & Febiger, 1988.

Turgeon ML: *Clinical Hematology: Theory and Procedures*, ed. 2. Boston, Little, Brown, & Company, 1993.

The book explores all major aspects of clinical hematology by dividing the information into an erythrocyte section, a leukocyte section, and a hemostasis section. Each section is further subdivided into chapter outlines that organize study material. At the end of each section, worksheets provide opportunities to focus on important concepts and definitions, sharpen calculation and problem-solving skills, and assess areas in which further study is needed. Different question formats are included for students with different learning styles. Multiple choice questions furnish a chance to test comprehension of the material. Answers with references to the above textbooks are included. The book also concludes with a comprehensive examination, also with answers and references, which challenges the student in much the same way as a national board examination.

A Study Guide of Clinical Hematology: Theory and Practice is not intended to replace the clinical hematology textbook. Instead, it should serve as a companion to the students' textbooks. Likewise, the study guide is not intended to be used by instructors in lieu of their own tests, for only instructors know what material is pertinent for their classes. Instead, it should serve as a tool to prepare the student to take different types of tests designed by the instructor.

We suggest that the student begin by looking at the chapter outlines for one section and studying the referenced pages in one of the textbooks. References are designated by the author's last name and are placed at the end of each outline. After studying the referenced material, the student should complete the worksheet for that section, check their answers, and review the references, which are placed beside the answer, for incorrect answers. Then, the student should proceed to the multiple choice questions for that section, check the answers, and once again review the references for incorrect answers. When working the multiple choice questions, the student should be careful to mask the answers using the page marker inserted in the book.

Every effort has been made to cite the best and most complete references; however, not all sources completely cover all topics. If the student's textbook does not adequately address the subject, the other references may provide additional insights.

When all sections have been completed, the student may assess total retention by taking the comprehensive examination. Once again, references are provided for each answer.

Janice L. Hudson
Robert F. Bunting, Jr.

Acknowledgments

We wish to acknowledge the contributions and encouragements we have received. Nadia D. Voss provided the idea for the study guide. The pathologists and hematology staffs of The Medical Center, St. Francis Hospital, and Martin Army Hospital contributed to histograms and photographs. We also thank our colleagues at Columbus College for their support. Our editor, Jean-François Vilain, and reviewers, Sally S. Greenbeck, Denise M. Harmening, and Sharon M. Kutt, suggested helpful changes and additions. We extend our deep appreciation to all.

Contents

— 🦌 —

Section One

——— ❧ ———

ERYTHROCYTES

Objectives for Erythrocyte Section

After studying the referenced material for each red blood cells (RBCs) chapter outline, completing the worksheet, and taking the section test, the student will be able to:

1 Describe normal RBC morphology

2 Evaluate and classify abnormal RBC morphology

3 Recall the composition of RBC inclusions

4 Explain the common causes of abnormal RBC morphology

5 Compare and contrast intravascular and extravascular hemolysis (catabolism)

6 State the globin chain composition of normal hemoglobins and common abnormal hemoglobins

7 Recall percentages of hemoglobin types that are present in the fetus, normal adult, and the adult with an abnormal hemoglobin

8 List the RBC metabolic pathways and their functions

9 State the role of albumin, haptoglobin, hemopexin, and transferrin

10 Describe normal RBC membrane, cytoplasm, and nuclear structure and function

11 Explain the ontogeny of hematopoiesis

12 Differentiate the stages of erythroid development

13 Demonstrate common sites used for bone marrow biopsies and aspirations

14 Calculate reticulocyte counts, corrected reticulocyte counts, reticulocyte production indices, absolute reticulocyte counts, myeloid to erythroid ratios, RBC indices, and manual RBC counts

15 Choose appropriate stains for confirmation of Heinz bodies and iron inclusions

16 State disorders in which RBC abnormalities are seen

17 Troubleshoot common specimen problems such as rouleaux, RBC agglutination, increased glucose, morphologic artifacts, and poor staining

18 Identify the effects of age, gender, and environment on hemoglobin levels

19 Classify anemias according to morphologic characteristics and cause

20 Evaluate laboratory data and choose a probable diagnosis

21 Distinguish among transferrin, ferritin, hemosiderin, and siderotic granules

22 Judge whether laboratory results pertaining to RBCs are normal

23 Distinguish between polycythemia and anemia

24 State the purpose of the following laboratory tests:

Acid elution stain	Complete blood count
Acidified serum lysis test/Ham's test	Donath-Landsteiner test
Antibodies to intrinsic factor	Erythrocyte sedimentation rate
Antiglobulin test—direct and indirect	Fluorescent spot test
Autohemolysis test	Free erythrocyte protoporphyrin
Bone marrow aspiration and biopsy	Haptoglobin

Heat denaturation test
Hemoglobin A_2 quantitation
Hemoglobin electrophoresis
Hemoglobin F quantitation
Iron studies
Methemoglobin assay
Osmotic fragility test
Plasma hemoglobin
RBC folate

RBC histograms
Reticulocyte count
Schilling test
Serum B_{12}
Serum folate
Sickle solubility test
Sugar water test/sucrose hemolysis test
Urine hemoglobin
Urine hemosiderin

Chapter 1

Hematopoiesis

I. Hematology
  A. The study of the concentration of cells in the blood
  B. The assessment of blood cell precursors
  C. The examination of the structure and function of blood cells
  D. The study of the role of vessels, platelets, and coagulation factors in hemostasis

II. Anticoagulants commonly used for blood specimens
  A. Ethylenediaminetetraacetic acid (EDTA)
    1. Mechanism of action: Binds calcium
    2. Uses
      a. Cell counts
      b. Morphologic examination
    3. Cautions
      a. Blood smears must be prepared within 2 hours of collection.
      b. Platelet clumping may occur in vitro.
  B. Sodium citrate
    1. Mechanism of action: Binds calcium.
    2. Use: Coagulation studies.
    3. Caution: Blood to anticoagulant ratio of 9:1 is important for accurate testing.
  C. Heparin
    1. Mechanism of action: Inhibits the action of thrombin.
    2. Use: Special hematologic testing.
    3. Caution: Heparin distorts cellular morphology and interferes with coagulation studies; therefore, its use is limited in hematology.

III. Hematopoiesis
  A. Definition: Production and maturation of blood cells
  B. Theory of cell origin
    1. A pluripotential stem cell is the precursor to all blood cell lines, including RBCs, white blood cells (WBCs), and platelets.
    2. Various factors influence development.
      a. Colony-stimulating factors (CSFs) are specific for various cell lines.
        (1) GM-CSF stimulates proliferation of granulocytes and macrophages.
        (2) G-CSF stimulates proliferation and enhances the function of neutrophils.
        (3) M-CSF stimulates proliferation of the macrophage-monocyte cell line.
        (4) Meg-CSF stimulates proliferation of megakaryocytes.
      b. Erythropoietin regulates proliferation of RBCs.
      c. Thrombopoietin regulates proliferation of platelets.
      d. Interleukins work in concert with CSFs to stimulate WBC production and maturation.
  C. Ontogeny
    1. The yolk sac is the earliest site of hematopoiesis, producing cells from the first weeks of embryonic life until 2 to 3 months gestation.
    2. The liver and spleen are the primary sites of hematopoiesis from 2 to 7 months gestation. This is known as extramedullary hematopoiesis.
    3. The lymph nodes are active throughout life starting at 4 months gestation.
    4. The bone marrow becomes the primary hematopoietic site from 7 months gestation throughout life. This is known as medullary hematopoiesis.
      a. Red marrow is the site within the bone marrow that produces the cells. In children the marrow in both long bones and flat bones is active, but in adults hematopoiesis occurs mainly in the flat bones.
      b. Yellow marrow is composed of fat and does not produce blood cells.

IV. Evaluation of hematopoiesis by bone marrow biopsy and aspirate
  A. Common aspiration sites

1. Infants: Proximal tibia
2. Adults: Posterior iliac crest, sternum, and anterior iliac crest

B. Evaluation
1. Myeloid:erythroid (M:E) ratio: Normally 2:1 to 4:1. The ratio is calculated by dividing the total number of granulocytes and their precursors by the total number of nucleated RBCs.
2. Cellularity: Evaluated by the fat cell to nucleated hematopoietic cell ratio.

3. Iron content: Iron in macrophages, nucleated red blood cells (NRBCs), and non-nucleated RBCs is estimated.
4. Differential: A specified number of nucleated cells are classified.

REFERENCES

Harmening: 24–27, 42–52
Lotspeich-Steininger: 18, 46–51, 366–377
McKenzie: 11–23, 100–102
Turgeon: 2, 16–17, 26–27, 44–51, 356

Chapter 2

Red Blood Cells and Laboratory Evaluation

I. Maturation sequence of RBCs in the bone marrow
   A. Rubriblast (pronormoblast): The size of the earliest recognizable precursor ranges from 12 to 21 micrometers in diameter. It has a large round nucleus with finely dispersed chromatin clumps and strands. Nucleoli are usually visible. The scant cytoplasm is dark blue due to the presence of ribonucleic acid (RNA). Numerous mitochondria and a prominent Golgi body are seen as clear areas in the cytoplasm.
   B. Prorubricyte (basophilic normoblast): The size varies from 11 to 17 micrometers. Nuclear chromatin is more clumped, yielding a smaller nucleus than in the previous stage. The cytoplasm remains dark blue. Nucleoli are present but may not always be visible.
   C. Rubricyte (polychromatophilic normoblast): The size varies from 11 to 14 micrometers. The nucleus acquires a "checkerboard" appearance with areas of densely clumped chromatin. The increased production of hemoglobin and the decreased production of RNA cause the cytoplasm to assume a gray color.
   D. Metarubricyte (orthochromatic normoblast): The size varies from 8 to 11 micrometers. The nuclear chromatin is extremely condensed and pyknotic. The decreasing prominence of ribosomal RNA, mitochondria, and the Golgi body allows the cytoplasm to stain bluish-pink. These cells are not normally seen in the peripheral blood of adults; however, a few may be present in newborns.
   E. Reticulocyte (diffusely basophilic erythrocyte): The size varies from 8 to 10 micrometers. No nucleus is present at this stage. Residual RNA remains in the cytoplasm resulting in a bluish-pink bi-concave disc.
   F. Erythrocyte (discocyte): The size varies from 6 to 8 micrometers. The mature RBC appears as a pink bi-concave disc as a result of the disappearance of RNA and the appearance of hemoglobin as the main cytoplasmic component (see figure on p. 10).

II. Maturation sequence of RBCs in the peripheral blood
   A. Reticulocyte (diffusely basophilic erythrocyte): This stage is normally the first stage released from the marrow. Reticulocytes comprise approximate 1 percent of the total peripheral RBC count and are seen on Wright's-stained smears as polychromasia.
   B. Erythrocyte (discocyte): The majority of RBCs in the peripheral blood are mature cells with a normal life-span of about 120 days.

III. Regulation of erythropoiesis
   A. Erythropoietin (EPO): The hormone is produced by the kidney in response to tissue hypoxia. As EPO increases, the bone marrow is stimulated to produce and release increased amounts of RBCs. When the RBC count reaches normal, the kidney reduces the amount of EPO produced which, in turn, decreases erythropoiesis.
   B. Androgens and thyroid hormones: These hormones enhance erythropoiesis.

IV. RBC synthesis and metabolism: Areas crucial to RBC survival and function
   A. RBC membrane
      1. Lipids: The membrane is a phospholipid bi-layer combined with glycolipids and cholesterol. Anions are freely permeable, but the cation pump is required for cation transport.
      2. Proteins
         a. Integral proteins, predominantly gly-

cophorin, span the lipid bi-layer acting as sites for RBC antigen formation.

b. Peripheral proteins, predominantly spectrin and actin, constitute a skeleton of microfilaments which control bi-concavity and deformability of the RBC. The ability to readily change shape and then resume the bi-concave disc is essential for the RBC to traverse the microcirculation.

B. Hemoglobin
   1. Synthesis and structure.
      a. Heme: Porphyrin rings are formed in the RBC cytoplasm and mitochondria, and then iron is incorporated into the molecule. Transferrin carries iron from the bone marrow hemosiderin stores to the RBC. Excess iron is deposited in the RBC cytoplasm as ferritin.
      b. Globin: At various stages of life, cytoplasmic ribosomes form six different amino acid chains—alpha (α), beta (β), gamma (γ), delta (δ), epsilon (ϵ), and zeta (ζ).
      c. Two globin dimers are joined to the heme molecule to produce hemoglobin.
      d. Normal hemoglobin molecules
         (1) Gower 1 ($\zeta_2\epsilon_2$): An embryonic hemoglobin generally present before birth.
         (2) Gower 2 ($\alpha_2\epsilon_2$): An embryonic hemoglobin generally present before birth.
         (3) Portland ($\zeta_2\gamma_2$): An embryonic hemoglobin generally present before birth.
         (4) F ($\alpha_2\gamma_2$): A fetal hemoglobin generally composing 55 to 80 percent of hemoglobin in the newborn. It rapidly declines to less than 2 percent of the total hemoglobin by 6 months of age.
         (5) A ($\alpha_2\beta_2$): A primary adult hemoglobin composing 95 to 98 percent of the total hemoglobin by 6 months of age.
         (6) A$_2$ ($\alpha_2\delta_2$): A secondary adult hemoglobin composing 1.8 to 3.5 percent of the total hemoglobin.
   2. Function: The transport of gases is influenced by pH, the 2,3-diphosphoglycerate (2,3-DPG) level, and the valence of iron.
   3. Influencing factors.
      a. Age
      b. Gender
      c. Geographic altitude
   4. Hemoglobin pigments.
      a. Oxyhemoglobin: Iron attached to the hemoglobin molecule is in the ferrous (Fe^{2+}) state with oxygen attached.
      b. Deoxyhemoglobin: Iron attached to the hemoglobin molecule is in the ferrous (Fe^{2+}) state but is not carrying oxygen.
      c. Carboxyhemoglobin: Hemoglobin molecule carries carbon monoxide.
      d. Methemoglobin: Iron attached to the hemoglobin molecule is in the ferric (Fe^{3+}) state.
      e. Sulfhemoglobin: Hemoglobin has irreversibly reacted with sulfur compounds. This pigment is not measured by conventional hemoglobin techniques.

C. Metabolism
   1. Embden-Meyerhof glycolytic pathway: Anaerobic glycolysis provides 90 percent of the RBCs' adenosine triphosphate (ATP) requirements.
   2. Hexose monophosphate shunt: Aerobic glycolysis is responsible for 5 to 10 percent of glucose utilization. It also protects the RBC from accumulation of hydrogen peroxide which denatures hemoglobin.
   3. Methemoglobin reductase pathway: The system maintains iron in the ferrous (Fe^{2+}) state which is required for oxygen transport.
   4. Luebering-Rapoport shunt: The pathway accumulates 2,3-DPG, which regulates oxygen delivery to the tissues.

V. RBC catabolism
   A. Extravascular hemolysis: RBC destruction by macrophage engulfment accounts for removal of 90 percent of aging RBCs. The heme and globin portions of hemoglobin are separated. Heme is further divided into iron, which is recycled, and porphyrin rings, which are eliminated as bilirubin. Globin is dismantled into amino acids which are returned to the amino acid pool.
   B. Intravascular hemolysis: RBC destruction by cell lysis within the vessel accounts for removal of 5 to 10 percent of aging RBCs. Free hemoglobin is complexed with available haptoglobin and removed by the liver. Residual free hemoglobin is excreted into the urine or converted to metheme. Metheme is then bound to hemopexin for catabolism in

the liver or bound by albumin to form met-hemalbumin, which remains in circulation until more hemopexin is made.

VI. Routine laboratory evaluation of RBCs
  A. Examination of the Wright's-stained peripheral blood smear.
    1. RBC size: 6 to 8 micrometers or the size of the nucleus of a small lymphocyte
    2. RBC shape: Round to slightly oval
    3. RBC color: Pinkish-orange with one-third central pallor
  B. RBC count.
    1. Manual
      a. Equipment
        (1) Neubauer hemacytometer
        (2) RBC pipet
      b. Diluting fluids
        (1) Gower's
        (2) Hayem's
        (3) Isotonic saline
    2. Automated
      a. Voltage pulse counting
      b. Light scatter
      c. Cell conductivity
  C. Hemoglobin (Hb).
    1. Colorimetric: Hemoglobin pigments are converted to cyanmethemoglobin and measured spectrophotometrically. As a rule, the value is 3 times the RBC count. Increased WBCs, lipemic plasma, or icteric plasma may interfere with colorimetric readings.
    2. Specific gravity: Hemoglobin is compared to a solution of known specific gravity.
  D. Hematocrit (Hct) (packed cell volume): As a rule, the value is 3 times the hemoglobin value.
    1. Manual: A capillary tube partially filled with blood is centrifuged and the percentage of RBCs is measured.
    2. Automated: The reading may be calculated from the mean RBC volume and the RBC count.
  E. Reticulocyte count.
    1. Manual: RNA within immature RBCs will precipitate with supravital stains. A specified number of RBCs are classified as mature RBCs or reticulocytes. Results may be reported as:
      a. Uncorrected count: Percentage of reticulocytes to total RBCs counted
      b. Corrected count: Uncorrected count multiplied by the patient's hematocrit divided by a normal hematocrit
      c. Reticulocyte production index (RPI): Corrected count divided by the maturation time of shift reticulocytes

      d. Absolute reticulocyte count: Total RBC count multiplied by the uncorrected percentage of reticulocytes
    2. Automated: Fluorescent staining can be used to tag RNA within the RBC. The fluorescence can then be evaluated by flow cytometer.
  F. RBC indices.
    1. Mean cell volume (MCV): Calculated average or directly measured average of the individual RBC volume. A normal MCV is termed normocytic; an elevated MCV is macrocytic; and a decreased MCV is microcytic. Spuriously increased results may occur in the presence of RBC agglutination, increased glucose, or elevated reticulocyte counts.

    $$MCV \text{ (in fL)} = \frac{\text{hematocrit (in L/L)}}{\text{RBC/L}}$$

    or

    $$\frac{\text{hematocrit (in \%)} \times 10}{\text{RBC/}\mu\text{L}}$$

    2. Mean cell hemoglobin (MCH): Calculated content of hemoglobin in the average RBC.

    $$MCH \text{ (in pg)} = \frac{\text{hemoglobin (in g/L)}}{\text{RBC/L}}$$

    or

    $$\frac{\text{hemoglobin (in g/dL)} \times 10}{\text{RBC/}\mu\text{L}}$$

    3. Mean cell hemoglobin concentration (MCHC): Calculated average concentration of hemoglobin in a volume of packed RBCs. A normal MCHC is termed normochromic; a decreased MCHC is hypochromic; and an elevated MCHC *usually* indicates false results.

    $$MCHC \text{ (in g/L)} =$$

    $$\frac{\text{hemoglobin (in g/L)}}{\text{hematocrit (in L/L)}}$$

    or

    $$\frac{\text{hemoglobin (in g/dL)} \times 100}{\text{hematocrit (in \%)}}$$

    4. RBC distribution width (RDW): Coefficient of variation of RBC volume.
  G. Erythrocyte sedimentation rate.
    1. Methods
      a. Wintrobe
      b. Westergren
      c. Zeta

2. Influencing factors
   a. Tube size
   b. Age and gender of the patient
   c. Protein level
   d. Anemia
H. RBC histogram: The normal RBC volume should follow a Gaussian curve with a mean between 80 and 100 femtoliters.

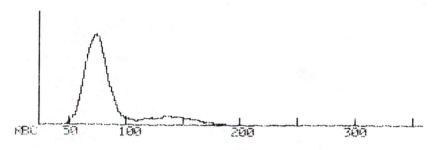

Femtoliters

REFERENCES

Harmening: 3–18, 27–30, 524–527, 530–536, 554–566
Lotspeich-Steininger: 27–29, 60, 63–64, 66–70, 72–84, 108–120, 234, 496–511
McKenzie: 25–29, 35–49, 85–90
Turgeon: 57–76, 307–315, 318–319, 325, 329, 339–343, 347–348, 350–354

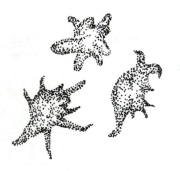

Acanthocytes

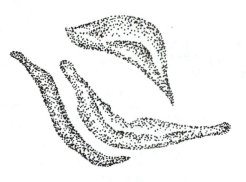

Drepanocytes (Sickle Cells)

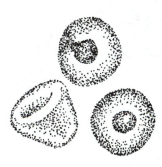

Codocytes (Target Cells)

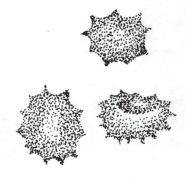

Echinocytes

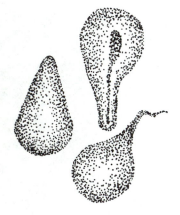

Dacryocytes (Teardrop Cells)

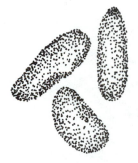

Elliptocytes

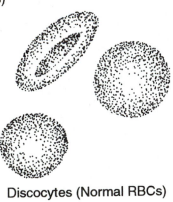

Discocytes (Normal RBCs)

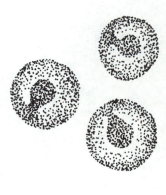

Leptocytes

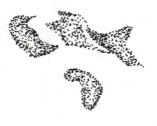

Shizocytes (Schistocytes)

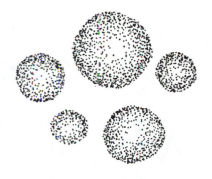

Anisocytosis

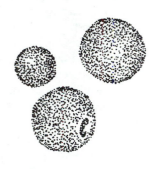

Spherocytes

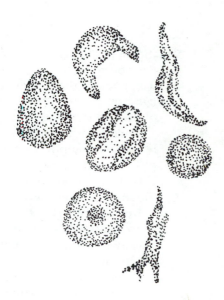

Poikilocytosis

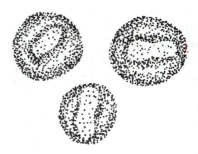

Stomatocytes

Chapter 3

Abnormal Red Blood Cell Morphology

I. Variations in RBC shape (poikilocytosis) and size (anisocytosis)

A. Acanthocyte, thorn cell, or spur cell (see figure on p. 10)
1. Description: A few irregular spines protrude from the RBC.
2. Common implications.
   a. Abetalipoproteinemia
   b. Liver disorders

B. Codocyte or target cell (see figure on p. 10)
1. Description: The RBC shows hemoglobin concentrations at the outer rim and center of the cell. A pale circular zone separates the two areas.
2. Common implications.
   a. Hemoglobinopathies
   b. Liver disorders
   c. Iron deficiency

C. Dacryocyte or teardrop cell (see figure on p. 10)
1. Description: The RBC is elongated but rounded on one end and pointed on the other end.
2. Common implications.
   a. Myeloproliferative disease
   b. Pernicious anemia

D. Drepanocyte or sickle cell (see figure on p. 10)
1. Description: The RBC is elongated with pointed projections on either end. The cell may be straight or curved.
2. Common implication: Sickling hemoglobins such as S, C Harlem, and I.

E. Echinocyte or crenated cell (see figure on p. 10)
1. Description: Regularly spaced bumps protrude from the RBC surface.
2. Common implication: The cells have been exposed to the anticoagulant for a prolonged period of time.

F. Elliptocyte or ovalocyte (see figure on p. 10)
1. Description: The RBC has bi-polar aggregates of hemoglobin that cause the cell to be slightly to severely elongated instead of round.
2. Common implications.
   a. Hereditary elliptocytosis
   b. Thalassemia
   c. Sickle cell anemia

G. Keratocyte, burr cell, helmet cell, or blister cell
1. Description: The RBC has extreme poikilocytosis with variable numbers of spines and spurs projecting from the membrane.
2. Common implication: Disseminated intravascular coagulation.

H. Knizocyte or triangle cell
1. Description: The RBC looks pinched into a triangular shape.
2. Common implication: Hemolytic anemia.

I. Leptocyte (see figure on p. 10)
1. Description: The RBC resembles a codocyte but is thinner yielding a small rim of hemoglobin at the edge of the cell.
2. Common implications.
   a. Iron deficiency
   b. Liver disorders
   c. Thalassemia

J. Macrocyte
1. Description: The diameter or volume of the RBC is larger than normal.
2. Common implications.
   a. B_{12} deficiency
   b. Folate deficiency
   c. Alcoholism
   d. Chemotherapy
   e. Reticulocytosis
   f. Spurious RBC size increase due to extremely elevated glucose levels

K. Microcyte
   1. Description: The diameter or volume of the RBC is smaller than normal.
   2. Common implications.
      a. Iron deficiency
      b. Thalassemia
      c. Anemia of chronic disease
      d. Sideroblastic anemia
L. Pyropoikilocyte
   1. Description: The RBCs are extremely variable in size and shape.
   2. Common implication: Hereditary pyropoikilocytosis.
M. Schizocyte or schistocyte (see figure on p. 11)
   1. Description: A piece of the RBC is missing causing the resultant RBC to appear fragmented and distorted.
   2. Common implications.
      a. Disseminated intravascular coagulation
      b. Mechanical trauma
N. Spherocyte (see figure on p. 11)
   1. Description: The RBC is round with no central pallor.
   2. Common implications.
      a. Hereditary spherocytosis
      b. Immune hemolytic anemia
O. Stomatocyte (see figure on p. 11)
   1. Description: The RBC is round with an elongated, mouth-like area of central pallor.
   2. Common implications.
      a. Hereditary stomatocytosis
      b. Alcoholism
      c. Artifact

II. RBC cytoplasmic inclusions
   A. Artifacts
      1. Description: Refractile areas and crenation in the RBC.
      2. Common implications.
         a. Water in the Wright's stain
         b. Poor staining technique
         c. Insufficient drying of slide prior to staining
   B. Basophilic stippling
      1. Description: Coarse granulation resulting from RNA aggregates. The granules are visible with Wright's stain and supravital stains.
      2. Common implications.
         a. Non-specific in anemias
         b. Lead intoxication
   C. Cabot rings
      1. Description: Thread-like round, oval, or figure-eight loops possibly due to resid-

ual nuclear membrane. The rings are visible with Wright's stain.
      2. Common implications.
         a. Pernicious anemia
         b. Lead intoxication
   D. Heinz bodies
      1. Description: Dark-staining round areas resulting from precipitated denatured hemoglobin. The bodies are visible with supravital stains but not with Wright's stain.
      2. Common implications.
         a. Glucose-6-phosphate dehydrogenase (G6PD) deficiency
         b. Heinz body anemias
   E. Hemoglobin C crystals
      1. Description: Oblong hexagonal crystals resulting from insoluble hemoglobin. The crystals are visible with Wright's stain and may be seen in combination with sickle cells.
      2. Common implications.
         a. Hemoglobin CC disease
         b. Hemoglobin SC disease
   F. Howell-Jolly bodies
      1. Description: Eccentric, small, round, non-refractile, purple masses consisting of deoxyribonucleic acid (DNA−nuclear remnant). The bodies are visible with Wright's stain and supravital stains.
      2. Common implications.
         a. Hemolytic anemias
         b. Post-splenectomy
   G. Parasites
      1. Description: Variable appearance depending on the parasite.
      2. Common implications.
         a. *Babesia* infestation
         b. *Plasmodium* infestation
   H. Porphyrin crystals
      1. Description: Needle-like, bluish rods consisting of non-heme porphyrin. The crystals are visible with Wright's stain.
      2. Common implication: Defect in porphyrin metabolism.
   I. Siderotic granules or Pappenheimer bodies
      1. Description: Small blue granules usually appearing in clusters near the periphery of the RBC and consisting of non-heme iron. The granules are visible with Wright's stain and can be confirmed by a Prussian blue stain. If the granules are in a NRBC, the cell is called a sideroblast. If the granules are in a non-nucleated RBC, the cell is called a siderocyte.
      2. Common implications.
         a. Post-splenectomy

  b. Sideroblastic anemia
  c. Sickle cell disease

III. Miscellaneous RBC Morphology
  A. Agglutination
    1. Description: Disorderly clumps of RBCs. If agglutination is due to cold agglutinins, clumps may be dispersed by warming the specimen.
    2. Common implications.
      a. RBC antibodies
      b. Autoagglutinins
  B. Anisocytosis (see figure on p. 11)
    1. Description: Variation in RBC size.
    2. Common implications.
      a. Anemia
      b. Transfusion therapy
  C. Hypochromasia
    1. Description: The central pallor of the RBC exceeds one third of the total cell size.
    2. Common implications.
      a. Iron deficiency
      b. Anemia of chronic disease
      c. Thalassemia
  D. Poikilocytosis (see figure on p. 11)

    1. Description: Variation in RBC shape.
    2. Common implications.
      a. Iron deficiency
      b. B_{12} deficiency
      c. Folate deficiency
      d. Hemolytic anemia
  E. Polychromasia
    1. Description: The cytoplasm of the non-nucleated RBCs has a grayish-blue tint.
    2. Common implication: Reticulocytosis.
  F. Rouleaux
    1. Description: Increased protein causes the RBCs to stack together like a roll of coins. Saline will disperse rouleaux.
    2. Common implications.
      a. Multiple myeloma
      b. Waldenström's macroglobulinemia

REFERENCES

Harmening: 67–73
Lotspeich-Steininger: 88–105
McKenzie: 91–100
Turgeon: 86–95

Chapter 4

Polycythemias and Non-hemolytic Anemias

I. Polycythemia
  A. Clinical symptoms
    1. Ruddy complexion
    2. Headaches
    3. Dizziness
  B. Relative polycythemia: An increase in RBC concentration due to a decrease in plasma volume
    1. Laboratory evaluation.
      a. RBC mass: Normal
      b. RBC count, hemoglobin, and hematocrit: Slightly increased
    2. Cause of acute cases: Loss of body water due to such episodes as vomiting, diarrhea, profuse sweating, or burns.
    3. Cause of chronic cases (Gaisböck's syndrome): Exact cause is unknown, but the plasma volume is low causing the RBCs to be concentrated in the peripheral blood.
  C. Absolute polycythemia: A true increase in RBC concentration
    1. Laboratory evaluation
      a. RBC mass: Increased
      b. RBC count, hemoglobin, and hematocrit: Increased
    2. Polycythemia vera
      a. Cause: Unknown
      b. Additional laboratory evaluation
        (1) Erythropoietin level: Normal to decreased
        (2) WBC and platelet counts: Often increased
    3. Secondary polycythemia
      a. Cause
        (1) Physiologic response to systemic hypoxia, such as chronic pulmonary disease, decreased oxygen at high altitudes, certain hemoglobinopathies, and massive obesity
        (2) Physiologic response to localized

renal hypoxia, such as obstructions and lesions which reduce blood flow to the kidney
        (3) Physiologic response to increased erythropoietin from some tumors
      b. Additional laboratory evaluation
        (1) Erythropoietin level: Normal to increased
        (2) WBC and platelet counts: Normal

II. Non-hemolytic anemias
  A. Iron disorders
    1. Clinical symptoms: Fatigue, shortness of breath, gastrointestinal disorders, skin pallor, and heart murmurs
    2. Classification
      a. Anemia due to iron depletion may be caused by:
        (1) Increased physiologic demand for iron during rapid growth, pregnancy, and increased hematopoiesis.
        (2) Increased loss of iron due to blood loss, hemolytic anemias, or cancer.
        (3) Malabsorption of iron due to gastrointestinal disorders.
        (4) Dietary deficiency. It is possible but not common in developed countries since the body efficiently recycles iron.
      b. Anemia of chronic disease due to the inaccessibility of storage iron: Disorders include autoimmune diseases, chronic renal failure, and cancer.
      c. Sideroblastic anemia due to the RBCs' failure to incorporate iron into the heme moiety.
    3. Laboratory evaluation
      a. Peripheral blood smear

        (1) Iron depletion: Microcytic, hypochromic RBCs with poikilocytosis.

        (2) Anemia of chronic disease: Normocytic, normochromic to microcytic, hypochromic RBCs.

        (3) Sideroblastic anemia: Dimorphic picture of microcytic, hypochromic RBCs and normocytic, normochromic RBCs. Siderocytes may be seen.

    b. Bone marrow iron stores

        (1) Iron depletion: Decreased to absent

        (2) Anemia of chronic disease: Increased

        (3) Sideroblastic anemia: Increased with ringed sideroblasts

    c. Hemoglobin: Decreased in all iron disorders

    d. RBC indices (MCV, MCH, MCHC): Decreased in all iron disorders

    e. RDW

        (1) Iron depletion: Increased

        (2) Anemia of chronic disease: Normal

        (3) Sideroblastic anemia: Increased

    f. Ferritin

        (1) Iron depletion: Decreased

        (2) Anemia of chronic disease: Normal to increased

        (3) Sideroblastic anemia: Increased

    g. Serum iron

        (1) Iron depletion: Severely decreased

        (2) Anemia of chronic disease: Decreased

        (3) Sideroblastic anemia: Increased

    h. Total iron binding capacity

        (1) Iron depletion: Normal to increased

        (2) Anemia of chronic disease: Decreased

        (3) Sideroblastic anemia: Normal to increased

    i. Percent iron saturation

        (1) Iron depletion: Severely decreased

        (2) Anemia of chronic disease: Decreased

        (3) Sideroblastic anemia: Severely increased

    j. Free erythrocyte protoporphyrin: Increased in all three iron disorders

B. Megaloblastic anemias

  1. Clinical symptoms: Skin pallor, weakness, dizziness, shortness of breath, slight jaundice, glossitis, weight loss, and epithelial aberrations

  2. Classification

    a. Anemia due to folate deficiency may be caused by:

        (1) Dietary deficiency

        (2) Malabsorption syndromes

        (3) Increased demand during pregnancy, neoplastic growth, and hemolytic crises

        (4) Drugs that act as folate antagonists

    b. Anemia due to vitamin B_{12} deficiency may be caused by:

        (1) Rare dietary deficiency

        (2) Malabsorption syndromes

        (3) Decreased intrinsic factor (pernicious anemia)

        (4) Increased demand during pregnancy, growth, parasitic infestation, and bacterial infection

  3. Laboratory evaluation

    a. Peripheral blood smear: Macrocytic, normochromic RBCs with oval macrocytes, anisocytosis, poikilocytosis, Howell-Jolly bodies, and polychromasia. Mature neutrophils may show hypersegmentation.

    b. MCV: Increased. This is not to be confused with falsely elevated results due to RBC agglutinins, extremely increased WBCs, elevated glucose levels, or reticulocytosis.

    c. MCHC: Usually normal.

    d. WBC and platelet counts: Decreased.

    e. Serum and RBC folate assays.

        (1) Folate deficiency: Decreased

        (2) B_{12} deficiency: Variable

    f. Serum B_{12} assay.

        (1) Folate deficiency: Normal or decreased

        (2) B_{12} deficiency: Decreased

    g. Lactic dehydrogenase: Increased.

    h. Gastric analysis.

        (1) Folate deficiency: Normal

        (2) B_{12} deficiency due to pernicious anemia: Achlorhydria

        (3) B_{12} deficiency due to malabsorption: Normal

        (4) B_{12} deficiency not due to pernicious anemia or malabsorption: Normal

    i. Schilling test.

        (1) Folate deficiency: Normal.

        (2) B_{12} deficiency due to pernicious anemia: Decreased without intrinsic factor supplement. Normal with intrinsic factor supplement.

        (3) B_{12} deficiency due to malabsorption: Decreased with and without intrinsic factor supplement.

(4) B_{12} deficiency not due to pernicious anemia or malabsorption: Normal.

j. Antibody to intrinsic factor.
  (1) Folate deficiency: Negative
  (2) B_{12} deficiency other than pernicious anemia: Negative
  (3) Pernicious anemia: Positive

k. Bone marrow biopsy and aspiration: Megaloblasts (large NRBCs with a webby chromatin pattern) are present. The cells show asynchrony in that the cytoplasm matures faster than the nucleus.

C. Aplasia and hypoplasia
  1. Acquired: Due to exposure of the bone marrow to toxins
  2. Hereditary: Fanconi's anemia
  3. Laboratory evaluation
    a. Peripheral blood smear: Pancytopenia
    b. Bone marrow aspirate: Aplasia to hypoplasia

REFERENCES

Harmening: 77–113, 346–361
Lotspeich-Steininger: 131–181
McKenzie: 109–125, 167–180, 185–191, 289–296
Turgeon: 58, 96–104, 229–233

Chapter 5

— ❧ —

Defects of the Red Blood Cell Membrane and Function

I. General laboratory findings following intravascular hemolysis (catabolism)
   A. RBC survival studies: Decreased
   B. Haptoglobin: Immediate decrease
   C. Methemalbumin: Increased for several days
   D. Urine hemosiderin: Increased for several days
   E. Plasma hemoglobin: Immediate increase
   F. Urine hemoglobin: Positive
   G. Bilirubin: Increased

II. General laboratory findings following extravascular hemolysis (catabolism)
   A. RBC survival studies: Decreased
   B. Serum unconjugated bilirubin: Increased
   C. Urine urobilinogen: Increased

III. Congenital membrane disorders causing hemolytic anemia
   A. Acanthocytosis
      1. Cause: Decreased plasma and membrane lipids result in irregularly formed RBCs.
      2. Additional laboratory evaluation
         a. Triglycerides and cholesterol: Decreased
         b. Peripheral blood smear: Marked acanthocytosis
         c. Reticulocyte count: Normal to increased
   B. Hereditary elliptocytosis
      1. Cause: Defective spectrin allows the RBCs to remain elliptical.
      2. Additional laboratory evaluation.
         a. Hemoglobin and hematocrit: Normal to severely decreased
         b. Peripheral blood smear: Elliptocytes
         c. Reticulocyte count: Slightly elevated
         d. Osmotic fragility: Variable
         e. Autohemolysis test: Variable
   C. Hereditary pyropoikilocytosis
      1. Cause: Defective spectrin results in variable RBC shapes and sizes.
      2. Additional laboratory evaluation.
         a. MCV: Decreased
         b. Osmotic fragility: Increased
         c. Peripheral blood smear: RBC budding, fragments, microspherocytes, and elliptocytes
         d. Heat sensitivity: RBC fragmentation when warmed to 45°C
         e. Autohemolysis test: Increased
   D. Hereditary spherocytosis
      1. Cause: A genetic defect prevents spectrin from functioning normally. The result is interference with RBC bi-concavity and deformability.
      2. Additional laboratory evaluation.
         a. Hemoglobin and hematocrit: Normal to moderately decreased
         b. MCHC: Usually increased
         c. Peripheral blood smear: Spherocytes and anisocytosis
         d. Reticulocyte count: Increased
         e. Osmotic fragility: Increased
         f. Autohemolysis test: Increased
   E. Hereditary stomatocytosis/hydrocytosis
      1. Cause: Defective cell permeability allows water to enter the RBC.
      2. Additional laboratory evaluation.
         a. MCV: Increased
         b. MCHC: Decreased
         c. Peripheral blood smear: Stomatocytes
         d. Osmotic fragility: Increased
   F. Hereditary xerocytosis
      1. Cause: Defective cell permeability allows water to exit the RBC.
      2. Additional laboratory evaluation.

a. MCV: Increased

b. MCHC: Increased

c. Peripheral blood smear: Codocytes (target cells) and RBCs with hemoglobin concentrated in one area of the cell

d. Osmotic fragility: Decreased

IV. Congenital metabolic disorders causing hemolytic anemia

A. Glucose-6-phosphate dehydrogenase (G6PD) deficiency.

1. Inheritance pattern: Sex-linked.

2. Cause: A decrease of G6PD in the hexose monophosphate shunt prevents synthesis of reduced glutathione. Reduced glutathione is required to prevent hydrogen peroxide buildup in the RBC during oxidant stress due to infections and certain chemical exposure. Increased levels of hydrogen peroxide irreversibly denature hemoglobin resulting in Heinz bodies. As RBCs with Heinz bodies traverse the microcirculation, hemolysis results.

3. Additional laboratory evaluation.

a. Reticulocyte count: Increased during hemolytic episodes

b. Supravital stain for Heinz bodies: Positive

c. Fluorescent spot test for G6PD: No fluorescence

d. Ascorbate-cyanide test: Positive

e. Quantitative G6PD assay: Decreased

B. Pyruvate kinase deficiency.

1. Inheritance pattern: Autosomal recessive.

2. Cause: A decrease of pyruvate kinase in the Embden-Meyerhof glycolytic pathway prevents synthesis of levels of ATP needed for adequate RBC function.

3. Additional laboratory evaluation.

a. Osmotic fragility: Normal

b. Incubated osmotic fragility: Often increased

c. Fluorescent spot test for pyruvate kinase: Decreased

d. Quantitative pyruvate kinase assay: Decreased

C. Methemoglobin reductase deficiency.

1. Inheritance pattern: Autosomal recessive.

2. Cause: A decrease of methemoglobin reductase in the Embden-Meyerhof glycolytic pathway allows hemoglobin to remain in the ferric (Fe^{3+}) state. The oxidized iron molecule cannot carry oxygen to the tissues.

3. Additional laboratory evaluation.

a. Methemoglobin assay: Increased

b. NADH-methemoglobin reductase activity: Decreased

D. Other enzymes in the Embden-Meyerhof glycolytic pathway and the hexose monophosphate shunt may be deficient. The deficiencies are rare and may cause hemolysis.

V. Paroxysmal nocturnal hemoglobinuria

A. Cause: An acquired structural or biochemical defect in the RBC, granulocyte, and platelet membranes causes the cell to be hypersensitive to complement. The sensitivity results in hemolysis.

B. Additional laboratory evaluation.

1. Reticulocyte count: Increased

2. RBC acetylcholinesterase: Decreased

3. WBC, RBC, and platelet counts: Decreased

4. Leukocyte alkaline phosphatase: Decreased

5. Urine hemoglobin: Positive in first morning urine

6. Sugar water test (sucrose hemolysis test): Positive

7. Acidified serum lysis test (Ham's test): Positive

8. Bone marrow biopsy and aspiration: Erythroid hyperplasia

REFERENCES

Harmening: 116–139, 183–190

Lotspeich-Steininger: 242–254, 262–265

McKenzie: 201–219

Turgeon: 71–75, 87–88, 104–107, 109

Chapter 6

Hemoglobinopathies

I. Quantitative disorders of globin chain production
  A. Hereditary persistence of fetal hemoglobin (HPFH)
    1. Cause: A congenital disorder prevents the "switchover" from gamma chains [hemoglobin F ($\alpha_2\gamma_2$)] to beta chains [hemoglobin A ($\alpha_2\beta_2$)].
    2. Laboratory evaluation.
      a. Hemoglobin: Normal
      b. Peripheral blood smear: Codocytes (target cells)
      c. Hemoglobin electrophoresis (cellulose acetate): Increased hemoglobin F and decreased hemoglobin A
      d. Kleihauer-Betke stain: Even distribution of hemoglobin F in all RBCs
      e. Alkali denaturation test for hemoglobin F: Increased
      f. Reticulocyte count: Normal
      g. Haptoglobin: Normal
  B. Thalassemias
    1. Alpha thalassemia
      a. Cause: A defect in one to four genes that control alpha chain production causes a mild to severe decrease in alpha chain synthesis depending on the number of genes affected. Since all functional adult hemoglobins consist of alpha chain dimers and a dimer of either beta, delta, or gamma chains, the decrease in alpha chains results in an excess of other dimers. The excess dimers then form tetramers that are nonfunctional.
        (1) Hemoglobin Bart's hydrops fetalis syndrome: The homozygous inheritance of the α^0-thalassemia gene creates a condition incompatible with life. Hemoglobin Bart's and hemoglobin Portland are predominant on electrophoresis.
        (2) Hemoglobin H disease: One alpha gene out of four is normal. Adults with this disorder have up to 40 percent hemoglobin H, which precipitates as golfball-like inclusions when the RBCs are incubated with brilliant cresyl blue.
        (3) α^0-Thalassemia trait: Two of four alpha genes are normal. The electrophoretic pattern is abnormal only at birth, showing up to 15 percent hemoglobin Bart's.
        (4) α^+-Thalassemia trait: Three of four alpha genes function. The electrophoretic pattern is abnormal only at birth, showing up to 2 percent hemoglobin Bart's.
      b. Laboratory evaluation.
        (1) Hemoglobin: Normal to severely decreased.
        (2) Peripheral blood smear: Codocytes (target cells) and microcytic, hypochromic RBCs.
        (3) Hemoglobin electrophoresis (cellulose acetate): Variable amounts of hemoglobin H (β_4) and hemoglobin Bart's (γ_4).
        (4) Brilliant cresyl blue stain: Hemoglobin H inclusions may be present.
    2. Beta thalassemia
      a. Cause: Mutant genes responsible for beta chain production cause decreased synthesis of beta chains. Since the predominant adult hemoglobin consists of two alpha chains and two beta chains, the decrease in beta chains results in alpha chain dimers. In an effort to compensate for the reduced normal adult hemoglobin A, hemoglobin F may increase.
        (1) Thalassemia major is a severe microcytic, hypochromic anemia resulting from the homozygous in-

heritance of the β^0-thalassemia gene (no beta chain production) or β^+-thalassemia gene (reduced beta chain production) or heterozygous inheritance of β^0 and β^+ genes.

    (2) Thalassemia intermedia is a milder anemia resulting from the homozygous inheritance of type 2 or type 3 β^+-thalassemia.

    (3) Thalassemia minor is a mild form of chronic microcytic, hypochromic anemia resulting from the heterozygous inheritance of a normal beta gene and a β^0- or β^+-thalassmia gene.

  b. Laboratory evaluation.

    (1) Hemoglobin: Normal to severely decreased depending on the severity of the genetic mutation.

    (2) Peripheral blood smear: Codocytes (target cells) and microcytic, hypochromic RBCs. NRBCs and basophilic stippling may also be seen.

    (3) Hemoglobin electrophoresis (cellulose acetate): Increase in hemoglobin A_2 and/or hemoglobin F.

    (4) Hemoglobin A_2 quantitation by ion exchange column: Increased.

    (5) Alkaline denaturation test for hemoglobin F: Slight to marked increase.

    (6) Kleihauer-Betke stain: Uneven distribution of hemoglobin F in the RBCs.

    (7) Reticulocyte count: Increased.

II. Qualitative disorders of globin chain production
  A. Hemoglobin S
    1. Cause: An autosomal mutation causes valine to be substituted for glutamic acid at the sixth amino acid position of the beta globin chain. The structural formula for homozygous inheritance is $\alpha_2\beta_2^{6glu \rightarrow val}$. The structural formula for heterozygous inheritance is $\alpha_2\beta_1\beta_1^{6glu \rightarrow val}$. The amino acid substitution produces a hemoglobin that crystallizes and is insoluble under low oxygen conditions. Heterozygous inheritance (sickle cell trait) results in minimal problems, while homozygous inheritance (sickle cell disease) creates severe difficulties.

    2. Factors that influence severity of the disease.
      a. Levels of hemoglobins S and F
      b. Availability of oxygen

      c. Presence of other hemoglobinopathies
      d. Dehydration
      e. Blood viscosity

    3. Types of crises.
      a. Aplastic: Temporary interruption of hematopoiesis
      b. Hemolytic: Increased RBC destruction
      c. Vaso-occlusive: Obstruction of blood vessels by sickled cells

    4. Laboratory evaluation.
      a. Hemoglobin
        (1) Sickle cell trait: Normal
        (2) Sickle cell disease: Decreased after 6 months of age
      b. Peripheral blood smear
        (1) Sickle cell trait: Codocytes (target cells) and rare drepanocytes (sickle cells).
        (2) Sickle cell disease: Codocytes (target cells), drepanocytes (sickle cells), ovalocytes, and polychromasia. NRBCs, siderotic granules, and Howell-Jolly bodies may be present.
      c. Sickle solubility test
        (1) Sickle cell trait: Positive
        (2) Sickle cell disease: Positive
      d. Hemoglobin electrophoresis (cellulose acetate)
        (1) Sickle cell trait: Approximately 60 percent hemoglobin A and 40 percent hemoglobin S. Hemoglobin A_2 may be slightly increased.
        (2) Sickle cell disease: At least 80 percent hemoglobin S. Hemoglobins F and A_2 may be slightly increased.
      e. Reticulocyte count
        (1) Sickle cell trait: Normal
        (2) Sickle cell disease: Increased

  B. S-beta thalassemia
    1. Cause: The individual is doubly heterozygous for thalassemia and hemoglobin S. The combination produces a disease similar to sickle cell disease.
    2. Laboratory evaluation.
      a. Hemoglobin: Normal to severely decreased
      b. Peripheral blood smear: Varies from slight anisocytosis to numerous codocytes (target cells) and drepanocytes (sickle cells)
      c. Sickle solubility test: Positive
      d. Hemoglobin electrophoresis (cellulose acetate): Predominantly hemoglobin S with variable amounts of hemoglobin A. Hemoglobins A_2 and F will be elevated.

e. Reticulocyte count: Normal to increased

C. Hemoglobin C

1. Cause: An autosomal mutation causes lysine to be substituted for glutamic acid at the sixth amino acid position of the beta globin chain. The structural formula for homozygous inheritance is $\alpha_2\beta_2^{6glu\rightarrow lys}$. The structural formula for heterozygous inheritance is $\alpha_2\beta_1\beta_1^{6glu\rightarrow lys}$. The amino acid substitution produces a hemoglobin that forms hexagonal crystals in the RBC. Heterozygous inheritance (hemoglobin C trait) results in minimal problems, while homozygous inheritance (hemoglobin C disease) creates more difficulties.

2. Laboratory evaluation.

   a. Hemoglobin
      (1) Hemoglobin C trait: Normal
      (2) Hemoglobin C disease: Decreased
   b. Peripheral blood smear
      (1) Hemoglobin C trait: Codocytes (target cells)
      (2) Hemoglobin C disease: Codocytes (target cells), hemoglobin C crystals, and folded cells
   c. Sickle solubility test
      (1) Hemoglobin C trait: Negative
      (2) Hemoglobin C disease: Negative
   d. Hemoglobin electrophoresis (cellulose acetate)
      (1) Hemoglobin C trait: Approximately 60 percent hemoglobin A and 40 percent hemoglobin C.
      (2) Hemoglobin C disease: At least 90 percent hemoglobin C. Hemoglobin F may be slightly increased.
   e. Reticulocyte count
      (1) Hemoglobin C trait: Normal
      (2) Hemoglobin C disease: Slightly increased

D. Hemoglobin SC

1. Cause: A combined inheritance of one mutant hemoglobin S gene and one mutant hemoglobin C gene creates moderate to severe clinical problems. Normal adult hemoglobin A is not produced.

2. Laboratory evaluation.

   a. Hemoglobin: Decreased
   b. Peripheral blood smear: Codocytes (target cells) and finger-like intracellular crystals
   c. Sickle solubility test: Positive
   d. Hemoglobin electrophoresis (cellulose acetate): Approximately equal amounts of hemoglobins S and C

e. Reticulocyte count: Increased

E. Hemoglobin D

1. Cause: A mutant gene causes glycine to be substituted for glutamic acid in the 121st amino acid position of the beta globin chain. The substitution creates no functional problems in heterozygous (hemoglobin D trait) or homozygous (hemoglobin D disease) states. Hemoglobin D may be confused with hemoglobin S on alkaline hemoglobin electrophoresis.

2. Laboratory evaluation.

   a. Hemoglobin
      (1) Hemoglobin D trait: Normal
      (2) Hemoglobin D disease: Slightly decreased
   b. Peripheral blood smear
      (1) Hemoglobin D trait: Normal
      (2) Hemoglobin D disease: Codocytes (target cells)
   c. Sickle solubility test
      (1) Hemoglobin D trait: Negative
      (2) Hemoglobin D disease: Negative
   d. Hemoglobin electrophoresis (cellulose acetate)
      (1) Hemoglobin D trait: Approximately equal amounts of hemoglobins A and D
      (2) Hemoglobin D disease: Approximately 95 percent hemoglobin D
   e. Reticulocyte count: Normal

F. Hemoglobin E

1. A mutant gene causes lysine to be substituted for glutamic acid in the 26th amino acid position of the beta globin chain. The substitution creates no problems in the heterozygous state (hemoglobin E trait) and minor problems in the homozygous state (hemoglobin E disease). Hemoglobin E may be confused with hemoglobins C and A_2 on alkaline hemoglobin electrophoresis.

2. Laboratory evaluation.

   a. Hemoglobin
      (1) Hemoglobin E trait: Normal
      (2) Hemoglobin E disease: Slightly decreased
   b. Peripheral blood smear
      (1) Hemoglobin E trait: Codocytes (target cells)
      (2) Hemoglobin E disease: Codocytes (target cells) and microcytes
   c. Sickle solubility test: Negative
   d. Hemoglobin electrophoresis (cellulose acetate)
      (1) Hemoglobin E trait: Approximately

equal amounts of hemoglobins A and E

    (2) Hemoglobin E disease: Approximately 95 percent hemoglobin E

  e. Reticulocyte count

    (1) Hemoglobin E trait: Normal

    (2) Hemoglobin E disease: Slightly increased

G. Hemoglobin M

  1. Cause: An amino acid substitution causes the hemoglobin iron to remain in the ferric (Fe^{3+}) form instead of the ferrous (Fe^{2+}) form. The ferric state cannot carry oxygen.

  2. Laboratory evaluation.

    a. Methemoglobin assay: Increased.

    b. Hemoglobin electrophoresis (cellulose acetate): Heterozygous inheritance produces approximately 30 percent hemoglobin M. Homozygous inheritance is incompatible with life.

H. Unstable hemoglobins

  1. Cause: Amino acid substitutions or deletions alter the configuration of hemoglobin. Hemoglobin then is easily denatured.

  2. Laboratory evaluation.

    a. Supravital stains for Heinz bodies: Variable

    b. Isopropanol precipitation: Positive

    c. Heat denaturation: Positive

REFERENCES

Harmening: 142–182
Lotspeich-Steininger: 185–229
McKenzie: 131–164
Turgeon: 67, 109–114

Chapter 7

Immune and Non-immune Hemolytic Anemias

I. General comments
  A. The indirect antiglobulin test (IAT) detects antibodies that have attached to RBCs in vitro. For example, if the patient is stimulated to produce antibodies to a foreign RBC antigen, these antibodies remain free in the plasma. When the patient's serum is incubated with reagent RBCs that have the corresponding antigen, the antibodies will attach to the reagent RBCs in the test tube. Anti-human globulin is then added to the cells. If antibodies have attached to RBCs, agglutination will occur indicating that antibodies are in the plasma. The IAT is positive in immune disorders and negative in non-immune disorders.
  B. The direct antiglobulin test (DAT) detects antibodies that have attached to RBCs in vivo. The patient must have both the antibody and its corresponding antigen present in the body at the same time for the test to detect the antibodies. When this occurs, the antibodies will attach to the RBCs while in circulation. When reagent anti-human globulin is added to a sample of the patient's cells, agglutination occurs indicating that antibodies are already attached to the cells. The DAT is positive for antibodies in autoimmune hemolytic anemia, transfusion reactions, and hemolytic disease of the newborn.

II. Immune hemolytic anemia
  A. Due to alloantibodies/isoantibodies
    1. Hemolytic disease of the newborn
      a. Cause: Fetal RBC antigens, if different from the mother's, may stimulate the mother to produce antibody against that antigen. If the antibody is IgG, it can cross the placenta and hemolyze the fetal RBCs. The most common antibody groups implicated in hemolytic disease of the newborn are ABO and Rh.
      b. Laboratory evaluation.
        (1) Maternal IAT
          (a) ABO: Variable
          (b) Rh: Positive
        (2) Fetal DAT
          (a) ABO: Variable
          (b) Rh: Positive
        (3) Fetal hemoglobin
          (a) ABO: Normal to slightly decreased
          (b) Rh: Moderate to severely decreased
        (4) Fetal bilirubin
          (a) ABO: Slightly increased
          (b) Rh: Increased
        (5) Peripheral blood smear
          (a) ABO: Spherocytes
          (b) Rh: NRBCs, anisocytosis, and poikilocytosis
    2. Hemolytic transfusion reaction
      a. Cause: An antibody that has been stimulated by a foreign RBC antigen will react with transfused RBCs carrying the same antigen. The reaction may be either immediate or delayed.
      b. Laboratory evaluation.
        (1) Urine hemoglobin
          (a) Immediate: Positive
          (b) Delayed: Negative
        (2) Haptoglobin
          (a) Immediate: Decreased
          (b) Delayed: Normal
        (3) Plasma hemoglobin

(a) Immediate: Increased
(b) Delayed: Normal
(4) Bilirubin
  (a) Immediate: Increased
  (b) Delayed: Increased
(5) IAT
  (a) Immediate: Positive
  (b) Delayed: Positive
(6) DAT
  (a) Immediate: Positive
  (b) Delayed: Positive

B. Due to autoantibodies
1. Warm autoimmune hemolytic anemia
  a. Cause: IgG autoantibodies may be of unknown origin or secondary to another autoimmune disorder such as lupus or lymphoma. The most common antibody specificity is anti-e. These antibodies react with the patient's own RBC antigens.
  b. Laboratory evaluation.
   (1) DAT: Positive
   (2) Hemoglobin: Decreased
   (3) Bilirubin: Increased
   (4) Peripheral blood smear: Spherocytes
2. Cold autoimmune hemolytic anemia
  a. Primary cold agglutinin disease
   (1) Cause: An unknown stimulus causes an elevation in a pathologic cold antibody, usually anti-I. These antibodies react with the patient's own RBC antigens.
   (2) Laboratory evaluation.
    (a) DAT: Positive.
    (b) Reticulocyte count: Increased.
    (c) Peripheral blood smear: RBC aggregates are seen unless the specimen is kept at 37°C until the smear is made.
  b. Secondary cold agglutinin disease
   (1) Cause: An infection triggers a transient increase in an autoantibody. The antibody is usually anti-I.
   (2) Laboratory evaluation.
    (a) Hemoglobin: Decreased
    (b) DAT: Positive
3. Paroxysmal cold hemoglobinuria
  a. Cause: A viral infection, usually in children, triggers production of anti-P, the Donath-Landsteiner antibody. The antibody causes hemolysis following exposure of RBCs to cold temperatures.
  b. Laboratory evaluation.
   (1) Donath-Landsteiner test: Positive
   (2) Urine hemoglobin: Positive
   (3) DAT: Positive during the hemolytic episode
4. Drug-induced immune hemolytic anemia.
  a. Cause: RBC hemolysis is triggered by one of several mechanisms in which the drug, RBC antigen, and a drug-related antibody interact.
  b. Laboratory evaluation
   (1) Plasma hemoglobin: Variable
   (2) DAT: Positive

III. Non-immune hemolytic anemia
A. Microangiopathic hemolytic anemia.
1. Cause: Changes in the microcapillaries traumatize RBCs causing shortened RBC survival. Diseases included in this category are disseminated intravascular coagulation, hemolytic uremic syndrome, and thrombotic thrombocytopenic purpura.
2. Laboratory evaluation.
  a. Hemoglobin: Normal to marked decrease
  b. Peripheral blood smear: Schistocytes
  c. Haptoglobin: Decreased
  d. Plasma hemoglobin: Increased
  e. Reticulocyte count: Increased
  f. DAT: Negative
  g. D-dimer: Increased
B. Parasitic infestation: The most common parasite to cause anemia is *Plasmodium*.
C. Miscellaneous mechanical damage.
1. Cause: Prosthetic heart valves, vigorous exercise, infections, or burns may create RBC fragmentation.
2. Laboratory evaluation.
  a. Peripheral blood smear: Schistocytes
  b. Plasma hemoglobin: Variable
  c. Urine hemoglobin: Variable

REFERENCES

Harmening: 193–211
Lotspeich-Steininger: 257–262, 267–278
McKenzie: 221–248
Turgeon: 107–109

Section One Worksheets

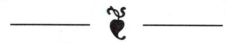

1. Identify the common sites of bone marrow biopsies and aspirations by writing the name of the bone next to the letters A, B, C, and D.

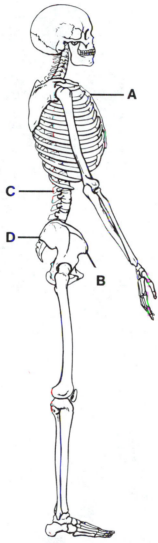

Adapted from Harmening DM: *Clinical Hematology and Fundamentals of Hemostasis*, ed 2. Philadelphia. FA Davis Company, 1992, p. 45, with permission.

2. Calculate the M : E ratio from the following bone marrow differential count of 500 cells.

Myeloblasts	10
Promyelocytes	20
Myelocytes	105
Metamyelocytes	180
Segmented neutrophils	80

Rubriblasts	0
Prorubricytes	10
Rubricytes	25
Metarubricytes	25
Lymphocytes	35
Plasma cells	5
Monocytes	5

3. Identify the following cells.

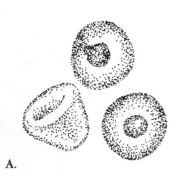 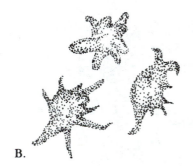 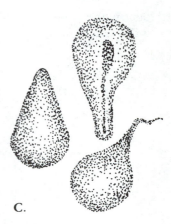

A.   B.   C.

4. Define the following:

    A. Peripheral (intrinsic) proteins

    B. Integral (extrinsic) proteins

    C. Globin

    D. Carboxyhemoglobin

    E. Methemoglobin

    F. Sulfhemoglobin

G. Extravascular hemolysis (catabolism)

H. Intravascular hemolysis (catabolism)

5. Identify three processes that are necessary for normal hemoglobin production.

6. Match the normal hemoglobins on the left with the appropriate polypeptide tetramers on the right. Each may be used only once.

A. _____ Hemoglobin A   a. $\alpha_2\delta_2$

B. _____ Hemoglobin A_2 b. $\zeta_2\epsilon_2$

C. _____ Hemoglobin F   c. $\alpha_2\beta_2$

D. _____ Hemoglobin Gower 1   d. $\alpha_2\epsilon_2$

E. _____ Hemoglobin Gower 2   e. $\alpha_2\gamma_2$

F. _____ Hemoglobin Portland   f. $\zeta_2\gamma_2$

7. Match the hemoglobins on the left with the normal percentages found in an adult. Answers may be used more than once or not at all.

A. _____ Hemoglobin A   a. 0%

B. _____ Hemoglobin A_2 b. <2%

C. _____ Hemoglobin F   c. 1.8–3.5%

D. _____ Hemoglobin Gower 1   d. 50–80%

E. _____ Hemoglobin Gower 2   e. 95–98%

F. _____ Hemoglobin Portland   f. 100%

8. State the function of each of the following RBC metabolic pathways.

A. Embden-Meyerhof pathway

B. Hexose monophosphate shunt

C. Methemoglobin reductase pathway

D. Luebering-Rapoport pathway

9. List the steps involved in **extravascular hemolysis** (catabolism)

10. List the steps involved in **intravascular hemolysis** (catabolism)

11. **Match the protein with the substance it carries. Each may be used only once.**

   A. _____ Albumin   a. **Bilirubin**

   B. _____ Haptoglobin   b. **Hemoglobin**

   C. _____ Hemopexin   c. **Iron**

   D. _____ Transferrin   d. **Heme**

12. **Label the following diagram with the appropriate globin chain. The choices are alpha chains, beta chains, gamma chains, delta chains, or epsilon and zeta chains.**

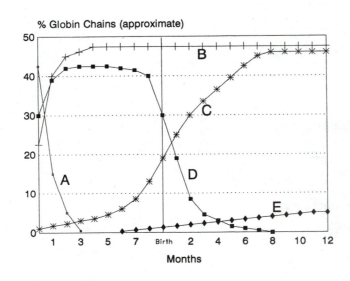

13. Define the following:

    A. Hematopoiesis

    B. Medullary hematopoiesis

    C. Extramedullary hematopoiesis

    D. Multipotential stem cell

14. List the organs or systems involved in hematopoiesis.

15. Name at least three features of the RBC that change as the cell matures.

16. List the stages of erythroid development from least mature to most mature. Use at least two different nomenclatures.

17. Identify the RBC from the following description on a Wright's-stained smear.

    A. The cell has pinkish-gray cytoplasm with a solid blue-black pyknotic nucleus.

    B. The cell has royal blue cytoplasm with a large round nucleus. The nucleus has visible nucleoli and no evidence of chromatin clumping.

    C. The cell contains no nucleus and the cytoplasm stains a pinkish color with a blue tinge.

    D. The cytoplasm of the cell has a bluish-pink color. The nucleus is coarsely clumped with no visible nucleoli.

18. Indicate whether the following statements are true (T) or false (F). If the statement is false, change the statement to make it true.

    A. _____ The blue color of the cytoplasm of immature cells is due to the abundance of DNA.

    B. _____ Nucleated RBCs may be seen in the blood of normal newborn infants.

    C. _____ The diameter of the normal mature RBC is about the same size as the nucleus of a small lymphocyte.

19. Identify three factors which influence the normal hemoglobin level.

20. Label the following diagram of a Neubauer hemacytometer with the appropriate size dimensions. In addition, identify the standard squares to be used for RBC counts and WBC counts.

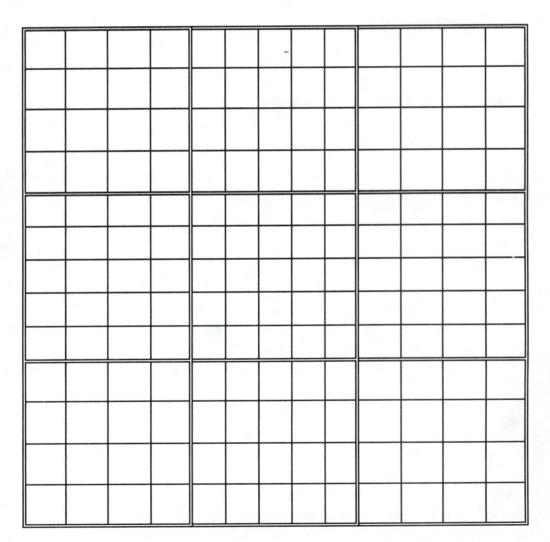

21. A. Blood is pipetted to the 1.0 mark of the RBC pipet, and the number of cells counted in the standard RBC squares equals 350 RBCs. Calculate the RBC count.

B. Is the value consistent with a normal adult female?

22. A. Blood is pipetted to the 0.5 mark of the RBC pipet, and the number of cells counted in the large center primary square on both sides of the hemacytometer equals 2400 RBCs. Calculate the RBC count.

B. Is the value consistent with a normal adult male?

23. State the formulas for calculating the following RBC indices.
   A. MCV

   B. MCH

C. MCHC

24. State the normal ranges for the following RBC indices.

    A. MCV

    B. MCH

    C. MCHC

25. Given the following patient data, calculate the MCV, MCH, and MCHC.

    A. WBC $= 7.0 \times 10^9$/L
       RBC $= 2.93 \times 10^{12}$/L
       Hb $= 81$ g/L
       Hct $= 0.235$ L/L

B. WBC = 10.3×10^9/L
   RBC = 1.95×10^{12}/L
   Hb   = 78 g/L
   Hct = 0.236 L/L

C. WBC = 3.8×10^9/L
   RBC = 3.32×10^{12}/L
   Hb   = 55 g/L
   Hct = 0.193 L/L

26. Describe the anemias that were calculated in the previous question. For example: normocytic, normochromic.

   A.

   B.

   C.

27. Calculate the RBC indices on patients with the following laboratory data.

    A. WBC = 7.5×10^9/L
       RBC = 4.91×10^{12}/L
       Hb　= 147 g/L
       Hct　= 0.440 L/L

    B. WBC = 3.4×10^9/L
       RBC = 2.15×10^{12}/L
       Hb　= 84 g/L
       Hct　= 0.240 L/L

28. A reticulocyte count reveals 305 reticulocytes per 1000 RBCs on a 6-year-old black male with sickle cell disease. The patient's RBC count is 2.95×10^{12}/L and the hematocrit is 0.270 L/L. Calculate the following values:

    A. Uncorrected reticulocyte count

B. Absolute reticulocyte count

C. Corrected reticulocyte count

D. Reticulocyte production index

E. Are the values consistent with the patient's disease state?

29. Use the data on each patient to make the requested calculations.
    A. 65-year-old male
       RBC = 2.56×10^{12}/L
       Hct = 0.232 L/L
       Number of reticulocytes seen per 1000 RBCs = 99

    Calculate the following:

    Uncorrected reticulocyte count

    Reticulocyte production index

Is this RPI consistent with a hemolytic state?

B. 17-year-old female
RBC = $3.78 \times 10^{12}/L$
Hct = 0.345 L/L
Number of reticulocytes seen per 1000 RBCs = 15

Calculate the following:

Uncorrected reticulocyte count

Reticulocyte production index

Is this RPI consistent with a hemolytic state?

30. Identify at least four factors that affect the erythrocyte sedimentation rate.

31. Describe the mature RBC.

32. Match the pathway on the left with the function of the pathway on the right.

    A. _____ Embden-Meyerhof pathway

        a. Synthesis of 2,3-DPG

    B. _____ Luebering-Rapoport pathway

        b. Majority of glucose utilization and ATP production

    C. _____ Methemoglobin reductase pathway

        c. Maintain the ferrous (Fe^{2+}) state of iron

    D. _____ Hexose monophosphate shunt

        d. Protects RBCs from environmental oxidants

33. Define the following:

    A. Anisocytosis

    B. Poikilocytosis

    C. Macrocytes

    D. Microcytes

34. Classify the predominant RBC morphology on the following photographs of Wright's-stained smears.

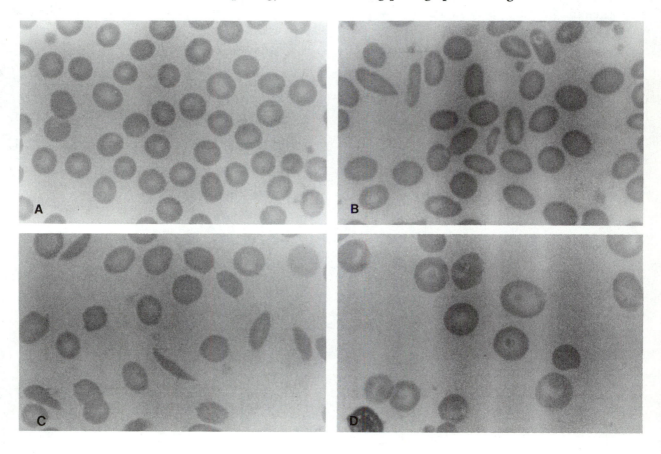

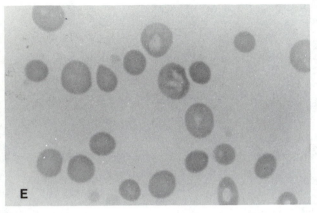

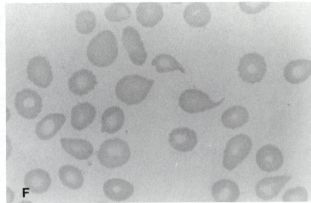

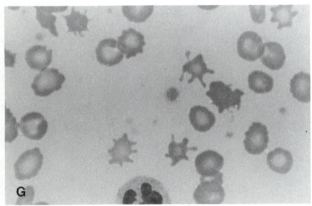

35. Match the RBC abnormality on the left with a disease state in which it is most commonly found. Use each letter only once.

A. ____ Schizocytes (schistocytes)	a. G6PD deficiency
B. ____ Howell-Jolly bodies	b. Porphyrias
C. ____ Basophilic stippling	c. Sideroblastic anemia
D. ____ Spherocytes	d. Sickle cell anemia
E. ____ Pappenheimer bodies	e. Paroxysmal cold hemoglobinuria
F. ____ Rouleaux	f. Disseminated intravascular coagulation
G. ____ Codocytes (target cells)	g. Multiple myeloma
H. ____ Heinz bodies	h. Abetalipoproteinemia
I. ____ Drepanocytes	i. Liver disease
J. ____ Dacryocytes (teardrop cells)	j. Severe burns
K. ____ Stomatocytes	k. Megaloblastic anemias
L. ____ Agglutination	l. Rh_{null} phenotype
M. ____ Acanthocytes	m. Myeloid metaplasia
	n. Lead intoxication

36. State the composition of each RBC inclusion.

A. Howell-Jolly bodies

   B. Basophilic stippling

   C. Siderotic granules

   D. Heinz bodies

   E. Cabot rings

37. Name at least three physical signs of anemia.

38. Place a "T" by the true statements and a "F" by the false statements. Correct the false statements.
   A. _____ The major source of the daily iron requirement comes from dietary iron absorption.
   B. _____ Iron requirements vary with age and gender.
   C. _____ A decrease in iron reserves should cause an increase in gastrointestinal mucosal absorption of iron.
   D. _____ The most common cause of iron deficiency anemia in postmenopausal women is gastrointestinal bleeding.
   E. _____ Anemia of chronic disease (inflammation) may be distinguished from iron deficiency anemia by the serum iron level.

39. Match the component on the left with the proper definition on the right. Each answer may be used only once or not at all.
   A. _____ Transferrin
   B. _____ Ferritin
   C. _____ Hemosiderin
   D. _____ Siderotic granules

   a. Water-insoluble iron storage compound
   b. Transport protein specific for iron
   c. Serum iron
   d. Major storage iron compound
   e. Iron inclusions

40. Interpret the following laboratory data for each of patients A, B, and C. Your choices are no anemia, iron deficiency anemia, anemia of chronic disease, or sideroblastic anemia.

Laboratory Test	Normal Range	Patient A	Patient B	Patient C
Hemoglobin (g/L)	Male: 135–180 Female: 120–160	Male 140	Female 70	Female 83
MCV (fL)	80–98	85.2	64.3	72.1
MCH (pg)	27–32	29.4	20.3	22.3
MCHC (g/L)	320–360	333	315	309
RDW (%)	11.5–14.5	12.5	19.1	12.9
Serum ferritin (μg/L)	Male: 20–270 Female: 16–150	150	5	150
Serum iron (μg/dL)	55–160	102	30	37
TIBC (μg/dL)	230–400	354	600	250
% Saturation	20–55	29	5	15
Free erythrocyte protoporphyrin (μg/dL)	17–77	48	200	150
Interpretation				

41. State at least two common clinical manifestations of vitamin B_{12} or folate deficiency.

42. Describe the typical peripheral blood smear morphology from a patient with megaloblastic anemia.

43. Define the following:

A. Megaloblast

B. Asynchrony

44. Name at least one patient condition that may lead to a falsely elevated MCV.

45. Interpret the following laboratory data by giving a probable cause of the macrocytosis for each of patients A, B, and C.

Laboratory Test	Normal Range	Patient A	Patient B	Patient C
Hemoglobin (g/L)	Male: 135–180 Female: 120–160	Male 70	Male 104	Female 60
MCV (fL)	80–98	123.2	103.2	115.3
MCH (pg)	27–32	40.2	33.0	38.9
MCHC (g/L)	320–360	327	320	338
RDW (%)	11.5–14.5	19.5	14.9	15.5
RBC morphology	Normocytic, normochromic	Oval macrocytes, Howell-Jolly bodies, anisocytosis, poikilocytosis	Macrocytes, polychromasia, anisocytosis	Oval macrocytes, Howell-Jolly bodies, anisocytosis, poikilocytosis
Reticulocyte count (%)	0.5–1.8	0.5	10.9	1.2
Serum B_{12} (pg/mL)	200–900	504	661	55
Serum folate (ng/mL)	2–16	1	11	7
RBC folate (ng/mL)	150–700	25	600	425
Anti-IF antibodies	Negative	Negative	Negative	Positive
Schilling test (% excretion)	>8	15	18	5
Interpretation				

46. Define the following:

    A. Aplastic anemia

    B. Fanconi's anemia

47. List two causative categories for aplastic anemia.

48. Differentiate between anemia of chronic disease or inflammation and iron deficiency anemia by completing the following chart of expected laboratory values. Use "↑" for increased, "↓" for decreased, or "nl" for normal.

Test	Anemia of Chronic Disease	Iron Deficiency Anemia
Serum iron		
Total iron binding capacity		
Ferritin		
Transferrin saturation		
Free erythrocyte protoporphyrin		
Storage iron		
Sideroblasts		
Reticulocyte production index		

49. Identify at least four causes of anemia of inflammation.

50. Explain why anemia develops when there is inflammation in the body.

51. Name two tests that are frequently used to establish the presence of hemolysis.

52. State whether the labeled osmotic fragility curves are increased or decreased resistance and name a condition in which each curve may be seen. The middle osmotic fragility curve is normal.

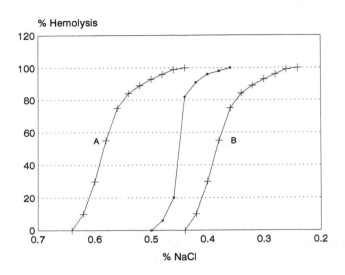

53. Fill in the parts of the chart that are not shaded. Identify the most common laboratory results for each hemolytic anemia listed.

Test	Hereditary Spherocytosis	Hereditary Elliptocytosis	Hereditary Pyropoikilocytosis	Hereditary Hydrocytosis	Hereditary Xerocytosis
Predominant RBC morphology					
Anemia					
MCV					
MCH					
MCHC					
Osmotic fragility					
Autohemolysis test					

54. Explain the possible inheritance patterns of G6PD deficiency.

55. Fill in the following chart with the typical results from a patient with PNH. Identify the principle or reason why the results are as stated. Skip any shaded box. The first test is completed as an example.

Test	Result	Principle
Acidified serum lysis test/Hams test	Normal to decreased	Highly sensitive RBCs lyse when exposed to complement
RBC indices		
Reticulocyte count		
RBC acetylcholinesterase		
Leukocyte count		
Leukocyte alkaline phosphatase		
Platelet count		
Urine hemosiderin		
Urine hemoglobin		
Indirect bilirubin		
Plasma hemoglobin		
Haptoglobin		
Direct antiglobulin test		
Sugar water test		
Acidified serum lysis tst/Ham's test		
Bone marrow aspiration and biopsy		

56. Discuss the cause of PNH.

57. Match the laboratory tests on the left with the results that would be expected to be present during an acute intravascular hemolytic episode. Answers may be used more than once or not at all.

A. _____ Haptoglobin   a. Normal

B. _____ Plasma hemoglobin   b. Increased

C. _____ Urine hemoglobin   c. Decreased

D. _____ Urine hemosiderin   d. Variable

E. _____ Bilirubin

58. If one parent is heterozygous for sickle cell (AS) and the other parent is homozygous (SS), what would be the inheritance pattern of the offspring?

59. State at least two factors that affect the severity of hemoglobin S.

60. Rank the following inheritance patterns from least affected by anemia to most affected: SS, AA, SC, AS, CC, DD.

61. Interpret the alkaline electrophoresis pattern for each of patients A, B, C, and D.

A.

B.

C.

D.

62. Interpret the following cellulose acetate electrophoresis (pH 8.4) by identifying the hemoglobins that are present and the most likely diagnosis (if appropriate) for each of patients A, B, C, and D.

A.

B.

C.

D.

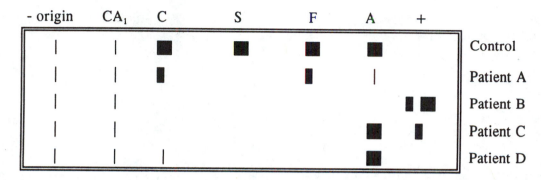

63. Define the following:

A. Aplastic crisis

B. Hemolytic crisis

C. Vaso-occlusive crisis

64. Match the disorder on the left with the appropriate category of abnormality on the right. Each letter may be used more than once or not at all.

A. _____ Beta-thalassemia

B. _____ Sickle cell disease

C. _____ Hemoglobin CC disease

D. _____ Beta-thalassemia sickle cell syndrome

E. _____ Alpha-thalassemia

F. _____ Hereditary persistence of fetal hemoglobin

G. _____ Hemoglobin Lepore syndrome

a. Structural abnormality

b. Rate of synthesis abnormality

c. Both a and b

d. Neither a nor b

65. Match the disorder on the left with the appropriate description on the right. Each letter may be used only once.

A. _____ Hydrops fetalis syndrome

B. _____ Hemoglobin H disease

C. _____ α^0-Thalassemia trait

D. _____ α^+-Thalassemia trait

a. Individual has hemoglobin Bart's at birth but develops a normal electrophoretic pattern later in life

b. Individual dies during gestation or soon after birth

c. Individual has no recognizable hemoglobin abnormality

d. Individual displays clinical symptoms of anemia but survives into adulthood without blood transfusion

66. Define the following:

    A. Alloimmune (isoimmune) hemolytic anemia

    B. Autoimmune hemolytic anemia

    C. Drug-induced hemolytic anemia

    D. Immediate hemolytic transfusion reaction

    E. Hemolytic disease of the newborn

67. Fill in the following chart with the expected results for each disorder. Use "↑" for elevated, "↓" for decreased, and "nl" for normal.

Anemia	RDW	Serum Iron	TIBC	Serum Ferritin	FEP	A$_2$ Level
Iron deficiency						
Alpha-thalassemia						
Beta-thalassemia						
Hemoglobin E disease						
Anemia of chronic disease						
Sideroblastic anemia						
Lead poisoning						

68. Match the laboratory test on the left with the purpose of the test on the right.

    A. _____ Direct antiglobulin test

    B. _____ Osmotic fragility test

    C. _____ Reticulocyte count

    D. _____ Hemoglobin electrophoresis

    E. _____ Fluorescent spot test

    F. _____ Iron studies

    a. To determine the response and potential of the bone marrow

    b. To evaluate storage and utilization of an essential mineral

    c. To detect the presence of immune globulin, complement, and their fragments/components

    d. To assess possible enzyme deficiencies

    e. To determine whether RBCs are more sensitive to lysis than normal

    f. To identify hemoglobinopathies and thalassemia syndromes

69. Identify the disorder causing hemolysis in each of patients A, B, C, D, and E. Choose from immune hemolytic anemia, G6PD deficiency, PK deficiency, methemoglobin reductase deficiency, hemoglobin M diseases, or enzyme deficiency not otherwise specified.

Laboratory Test	Patient A	Patient B	Patient C	Patient D	Patient E
Antiglobulin test	Negative	Positive	Negative	Negative	Negative
Osmotic fragility	Normal	Normal	Normal	Normal	Normal
Supravital stain for Heinz bodies	Negative	Negative	Positive	Negative	Negative
Fluorescent spot tet for G6PD	Fluorescence	Fluorescence	No fluorescence	Fluorescence	Fluorescence
Fluorescent spot test for PK	No fluorescence	Fluorescence	Fluorescence	Fluorescence	Fluorescence
Methemoglobin assay	Normal	Normal	Normal	Normal	Increased
Hemoglobin electrophoresis	Normal	Normal	Normal	Normal	Normal
Interpretation					

Answers to Section One Worksheets

1. A. Sternum

   B. Anterior superior iliac crest

   C. Spinal processes

   D. Posterior superior iliac crest

   REF: H:45; L:x; M:100; T:27

2. Total number of myeloid cells (myeloblasts, promyelocytes, myelocytes, metamyelocytes, segmented neutrophils) = 395
   Total number of nucleated RBCs (rubriblasts, prorubricytes, rubricytes, metarubricytes) = 60
   Ratio of myeloid cells to erythroid cells = 395 : 60 or 6.6 : 1
   REF: H:49 – 50; L:377; M:101; T:356

3. A. Codocytes (target cells)

   B. Acanthocytes

   C. Dacryocytes (teardrop cells)

   REF: H:72; L:93 – 95; M:93, 95; T:88

4. A. RBC membrane proteins that are on the membrane exterior. REF: H:4; L:66; M:28; T:33

   B. Those proteins in the RBC membrane that extend from the exterior to the interior of the cell membrane. REF: H:4; L:x; M:28; T:33

   C. Two dimers of polypeptide chains. REF: H:8; L:74; M:x, T:66

   D. Hemoglobin molecule carrying carbon monoxide. REF: H:14; L:83; M:45; T:67

   E. Hemoglobin molecule in which the iron is in the ferric (Fe^{3+}) state. REF: H:14; L:82; M:44; T:68

   F. Abnormal hemoglobin formed when the sulfur content of the blood increases. REF: H:14; L:83; M:45; T:68

   G. Removal of RBCs by phagocytic cells in the reticuloendothelial system. REF: H:16; L:234; M:46; T:74

   H. RBC destruction within the blood vessels. REF: H:17; L:234; M:46; T:74 – 75

5. Adequate iron transport and availability; adequate protoporphyrin production; adequate globin production
   REF: H:8; L:73; M:41; T:64 – 66

6. A. c

   B. a

   C. e

   D. b

   E. d

   F. f

   REF: H:9 – 10; L:73; M:83; T:66

7. A. e
    B. c
    C. b
    D. a
    E. a
    F. a
    REF: H:10; L:73; M:38; T:67

8. A. Provides 90% of the ATP required by RBCs
    B. Provides 5–10% of the ATP required by the RBC and neutralizes intracellular oxidants which denature hemoglobin
    C. Maintains heme iron in the reduced (Fe^{2+}, ferrous) functional state
    D. Causes accumulation of 2,3-DPG
    REF: H:15–16; L:67–68; M:30; T:72–73

9. RBCs are phagocytized. Hemoglobin is broken into components. Iron is returned to the bone marrow. Amino acids from globin chains are returned to the amino acid pool. Protoporphyrin ring is converted to bilirubin for ultimate excretion into the intestines where it is further converted to urobilinogen for excretion in the feces. Some urobilinogen is reabsorbed by the intestines and excreted in the urine. REF: H:16–17; L:234; M:197; T:74

10. RBCs rupture resulting in free hemoglobin dimers. Dimers form a complex with available haptoglobin. The complex is then broken down by the liver. Remaining hemoglobin dimers are excreted into the urine or converted to metheme. Metheme is bound by hemopexin for catabolism by the liver or bound by albumin to form methemalbumin, which remains in circulation until more hemopexin is available. REF: H:17–18; L:234; M:196; T:74–75

11. A. a
    B. b
    C. d
    D. c
    REF: H:18; L:234, 236; M:46–48, 112; T:74–75

12. A. Epsilon
    B. Alpha
    C. Beta
    D. Gamma
    E. Delta
    REF: H:12; L:213; M:x; T:66–67

13. A. Blood cell production and maturation. REF: H:22; L:46; M:11; T:44
    B. Blood cell production in the bone marrow. REF: H:22; L:438; M:11; T:44
    C. Production of hematopoietic cells in the spleen, liver, and tissues other than bone marrow. REF: H:23; L:438; M:11; T:46
    D. Uncommitted precursor cells that produce mature circulating blood cells which are committed to one cell line. REF: H:24; L:48; M:20; T:45

14. Bone marrow, liver, spleen, lymph nodes, thymus, and yolk sac. REF: H:22; L:47; M:11; T:44

15. Reduced cell volume; condensed nuclear chromatin; loss of nucleolus, then the nucleus itself; decreased cytoplasmic RNA; decreased mitochondria; increased hemoglobin
    REF: H:28; L:61–62; M:25; T:59

16. Rubriblast/pronormoblast/proerythroblast
    Prorubricyte/basophilic normoblast/basophilic erythroblast
    Rubricyte/polychromatophilic normoblast/polychromatic erythroblast
    Metarubricyte/orthochromatic normoblast/orthochromatic erythroblast
    Diffusely basophilic erythrocyte/polychromatophilic erythrocyte/reticulocyte
    Erythrocyte/discocyte/mature RBC
    REF: H:28–30; L:63; M:25; T:59

17. A. Metarubricyte

    B. Rubriblast

    C. Diffusely basophilic erythrocyte

    D. Rubricyte
    REF: H:28–29; L:64; M:26; T:58–60

18. A. F, The blue color of the cytoplasm of immature cells is due to the abundance of RNA. REF: H:29; L:64; M:26; T:58

    B. T, REF: H:29; L:48; M:x; T:x

    C. T, REF: H:36; L:x; M:67; T:x

19. Age; gender; geographic altitude
    REF: H:55; L:127; M:85–86; T:x

20.

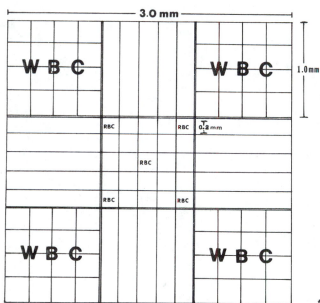

REF: H:524; L:318; M:x; T:340–341

Adapted from Harmening DM: *Clinical Hematology and Fundamentals of Hemostasis*, ed 2. Philadelphia. FA Davis Company, 1992, p. 45, with permission.

21. A.   Cells counted = 350
          Dilution = 1 : 100, therefore the reciprocal is 100
             Area = 0.2 × 0.2 × 5 = 0.2, therefore the reciprocal is 1/0.2 or 5
          Depth = 1/10, therefore the reciprocal is 10

    Actual cell count = 350 × 100 × 5 × 10
                      = $1.75 \times 10^6/mm^3$ or $1.75 \times 10^{12}/L$

    B. No

    REF: H:526; L:108, 318–319; M:x; T:339–341

22. A.   Cells counted $= 2400$

         Dilution $= 1 : 200$, therefore the reciprocal is 200

         Area $= 1 \times 1 \times 2 = 2.0$, therefore the reciprocal is ½ or 0.5

         Depth $= \frac{1}{10}$, therefore the reciprocal is 10

     Actual cell count $= 2400 \times 200 \times 0.5 \times 10$

                         $= 2.40 \times 10^6/mm^3$ or $2.40 \times 10^{12}/L$

B. No

REF: H:526; L:108, 318–319; M:x; T:339–341

23. A. $$\text{MCV (in fL)} = \frac{\text{Hct (in L/L)}}{\text{RBC/L}} \quad \text{or} \quad \frac{\text{Hct (in \%)} \times 10}{\text{RBC/}\mu\text{L}}$$

B. $$\text{MCH (in pg)} = \frac{\text{Hb (in g/L)}}{\text{RBC/L}} \quad \text{or} \quad \frac{\text{Hb (in g/dL)} \times 10}{\text{RBC/}\mu\text{L}}$$

C. $$\text{MCHC (in g/L or g/dL)} = \frac{\text{Hb (in g/L)}}{\text{Hct (in L/L)}} \quad \text{or} \quad \frac{\text{Hb (in g/dL)} \times 100}{\text{Hct (in \%)}}$$

REF: H:57; L:113–114; M:86–87; T:76

24. A. MCV is about 80–98 fL

B. MCH is about 27–32 pg

C. MCHC is about 320–360 g/L

REF: H:57; L:113–114; M:87; T:76

25. A. MCV $= 0.235 \div (2.93 \times 10^{12}) = 8.02 \times 10^{-14}$ L or 80.2 fL

MCH $= 81 \div (2.93 \times 10^{12}) = 2.76 \times 10^{-11}$ g or 27.6 pg

MCHC $= 81 \div 0.235 = 345$ g/L

B. MCV $= 0.236 \div (1.95 \times 10^{12}) = 1.21 \times 10^{-13}$ L or 121.0 fL

MCH $= 78 \div (1.95 \times 10^{12}) = 4.00 \times 10^{-11}$ g or 40.0 pg

MCHC $= 78 \div 0.236 = 331$ g/L

C. MCV $= 0.193 \div (3.32 \times 10^{12}) = 5.81 \times 10^{-14}$ L or 58.1 fL

MCH $= 55 \div (3.32 \times 10^{12}) = 1.66 \times 10^{-11}$ g or 16.6 pg

MCHC $= 55 \div 0.193 = 285$ g/L

REF: H:57; L:113–114; M:86–87; T:76

26. A. Normocytic, normochromic

B. Macrocytic, normochromic

C. Microcytic, hypochromic

REF: H:57; L:113–114; M:87; T:76, 87, 91–92

27. A. MCV $= 0.44 \div (4.91 \times 10^{12}) = 8.96 \times 10^{-14}$ L or 89.6 fL

MCH $= 147 \div (4.91 \times 10^{12}) = 2.99 \times 10^{-11}$ g or 29.9 pg

MCHC $= 147 \div 0.44 = 334$ g/L

B. MCV $= 0.24 \div (2.15 \times 10^{12}) = 1.116 \times 10^{-13}$ L or 111.6 fL

$$MCH = 84 \div (2.15 \times 10^{12}) = 3.91 \times 10^{-11} \text{ g or } 39.1 \text{ pg}$$

$$MCHC = 84 \div 0.24 = 350 \text{ g/L}$$

REF: H:532; L:113–114; M:86–87; T:76

28. RBC $= 2.95 \times 10^{12}$/L
Hematocrit $= 0.27$ L/L (normal range for 6-year-old males: 0.35–0.45 L/L)
Reticulocytes per 1000 RBCs $= 305$
Maturation time for hematocrit of 0.27 L/L $= 1.5$ days

A. Uncorrected reticulocyte count $= (305 \div 1000) \times 100 = 30.5\%$

B. Absolute reticulocyte count $= 30.5\% \times (2.95 \times 10^{12}$/L$) = 0.305 \times (2.95 \times 10^{12}$/L$)$
$= 0.8998 \times 10^{12}$/L $= 899.8 \times 10^9$/L

C. Corrected reticulocyte count $= 30.5\% \times (0.27 \div 0.40) = 20.6\%$

D. Reticulocyte production index $= 20.6\% \div 1.5 = 13.7\%$

E. Yes

REF: H:530–531; L:114–117; M:88–90; T:60–61

29. A. RBC $= 2.56 \times 10^{12}$/L
Hematocrit $= 0.232$ L/L (normal range for adult males: 0.40–0.54 L/L)
Reticulocytes/1000 RBCs $= 99$
Maturation time for hematocrit of 0.232 L/L $= 2.0$ days

Uncorrected reticulocyte count $= (99 \div 1000) \times 100 = 9.9\%$

Reticulocyte production index $= [9.9\% \times (0.232 \div 0.47)] \div 2.0 = 2.4\%$

This RPI is consistent with a hemolytic state.

B. RBC $= 3.78 \times 10^{12}$/L
Hematocrit $= 0.345$ L/L (normal range for adult females: 0.36–0.48 L/L)
Reticulocytes/1000 RBCs $= 15$
Maturation time for hematocrit of 0.345 L/L $= 1.5$ days

Uncorrected reticulocyte count $= (15 \div 1000) \times 100 = 1.5\%$

Reticulocyte production index $= [1.5\% \times (0.345 \div 0.42)] \div 1.5 = 0.8\%$

This RPI is not consistent with a hemolytic state.

REF: H:118; L:115, 117; M:89–90; T:60–61

30. Plasma proteins such as fibrinogen and immunoglobulins, type of anticoagulants used, anemia and poikilocytosis, specimen age and temperature, size and position of ESR tube
REF: H:534; L:118–119; M:x; T:352–354

31. Non-nucleated, bi-concave disc. It is pink with the middle one third having central pallor. The diameter varies from 6–8 μm and the average volume is 80–98 fL. REF: H:66; L:64; M:27; T:60

32. A. b
B. a
C. c
D. d
REF: H:136; L:67–68; M:30–33; T:72–73

33. A. Variation in the size of RBCs. REF: H:66; L:91; M:92; T:87

    B. Variation in the shape of RBCs. REF: H:66; L:92; M:92; T:87

    C. RBCs that are larger than normal (diameter > 9 μm, MCV > 98 fL). REF: H:66; L:90; M:96; T:87

    D. RBCs that are smaller than normal (diameter < 6 μm, MCV < 80 fL). REF: H:67; L:90; M:97; T:87

34. A. Discocytes. REF: H:72; L:89; M:27; T:88

    B. Ovalocytes (elliptocytes). REF: H:72; L:93; M:93; T:88

    C. Drepanocytes (sickle cells). REF: H:72; L:97; M:93; T:88

    D. Codocytes (target cells). REF: H:72; L:94; M:93; T:88

    E. Spherocytes. REF: H:72; L:92; M:93; T:88

    F. Dacryocytes (teardrop cells). REF: H:72; L:96; M:93; T:88

    G. Acanthocytes. REF: H:72; L:94; M:93; T:88

35. A. f. REF: H:70; L:95; M:95; T:x

    B. k. REF: H:71; L:98; M:98; T:93

    C. n. REF: H:71; L:98; M:98; T:92

    D. j. REF: H:68; L:x; M:94; T:91

    E. c. REF: H:71; L:99; M:99; T:93

    F. g. REF: H:71; L:89; M:360–362; T:93, 217

    G. i. REF: H:68; L:94; M:95; T:91

    H. a. REF: H:71; L:100; M:99; T:92

    I. d. REF: H:69; L:69; M:69; T:91

    J. m. REF: H:70; L:95; M:95; T:91

    K. l. REF: H:69; L:94; M:94; T:91

    L. e. REF: H:70; L:89; M:100; T:x

    M. h. REF: H:69; L:93; M:95; T:88

36. A. DNA/nuclear remnant

    B. RNA and mitochondrial remnants

    C. Iron

    D. Denatured hemoglobin

    E. Arginine-rich histone and non-hemoglobin iron

    REF: H:71; L:98–100; M:97–99: T:92–93

37. Weakness, fatigue, dyspnea on exertion, gastrointestinal disorders, pallor, mild temperature elevation, heart murmurs
    REF: H:56; L:127; M:84; T:x

38. A. F. The major source of the daily iron requirement comes from iron recycled from senescent RBCs. REF: H:81; L:77; M:110; T:99

    B. T. REF: H:80; L:174–175; M:115; T:99

    C. T. REF: H:81; L:77; M:111; T:99–100

    D. T. REF: H:84; L:175; M:116; T:x

    E. F. Anemia of chronic disease (inflammation) may be distinguished from iron deficiency anemia by the TIBC. REF: H:85; L:178; M:125; T:102

39. A. b. REF: H:80; L:78; M:112; T:99–100

    B. d. REF: H:81; L:77; M:110; T:36

C. a. REF: H:81; L:77; M:111; T:36

D. e. REF: H:79; L:98; M:98; T:93

40. A. No anemia

B. Iron deficiency anemia

C. Anemia of chronic disease

REF: H:85; L:173; M:125; T:99–102

41. Fatigue, dizziness, pallor, shortness of breath, slight jaundice, glossitis, weight loss, and epithelial abnormalities. REF: H:97; L:x; M:168; T:x

42. Oval macrocytosis, anisocytosis, poikilocytosis, Howell-Jolly bodies, basophilic stippling, Cabot rings, polychromasia, NRBCs, hypersegmented neutrophils, and pancytopenia. REF: H:98–99; L:157; M:168; T:104

43. A. Abnormally large NRBCs having immature-appearing, webby nuclear chromatic but normal-appearing cytoplasm. REF: H:92; L:158; M:x; T:x

B. The lack of coordination between nuclear and cytoplasmic maturation. REF: H:100; L:x; M:169; T:x

44. Cold autoagglutinins, elevated glucose level, reticulocytosis, and extremely elevated WBC count. REF: H:101; L:273; M:240; T:x

45. A. Folate deficiency. REF: H:101–104; L:159; M:173; T:104

B. Reticulocytosis. REF: H:101; L:236; M:181; T:61

C. Pernicious anemia. REF: H:101–104; L:161; M:178; T:104

46. A. A disorder in which hematopoiesis does not occur. REF: H:107; L:139: M:185; T:97–98

B. An autosomal recessive disorder that leads to progressive marrow aplasia and peripheral pancytopenia. REF: H:110; L:144; M:189; T:98

47. Acquired from toxic injury to the bone marrow, idiopathic and congenital. REF: H:108; L:139; M:187; T:98

48.

Test	Anemia of Chronic Disease	Iron Deficiency Anemia
Serum iron	↓	↓
Total iron binding capacity	↓	↑
Ferritin	↑	↓
Transferrin saturation	↓	↓
Free erythrocyte protoporphyrin	↑	↑
Storage iron	↑	↓
Sideroblasts	↓	↓
Reticulocyte production index	↓	↓

REF: H:225; L:173; M:117, 125; T:100–102

49. Infection, connective tissue disorders, malignancy, endocrine disease, renal disease, liver disease REF: H:225; L:178; M:124; T:101

50. Increased phagocytic activity by the macrophage-monocytes of the reticuloendothelial system may cause early RBC destruction. Iron is trapped in the macrophages of the reticuloendothelial system. Inadequate erythropoietin levels fail to stimulate RBC production. Suppression of erythropoiesis results from inhibitory effects of acute-phase reactants. REF: H:225–227; L:177–178; M:124; T:101–102

51. Serum unconjugated (indirect) bilirubin and serum haptoglobin
REF: H:116; L:234; M:102–103; T:74–75

52. A. Decreased osmotic fragility; hemoglobinopathies

    B. Increased osmotic fragility; hereditary spherocytosis or pyruvate kinase deficiency

REF: H:125; L:245; M:205; T:366–367

53.

Test	Hereditary Spherocytosis	Hereditary Elliptocytosis	Hereditary Pyropoikilocytosis	Hereditary Hydrocytosis	Hereditary Xerocytosis
Predominant RBC morphology	Spherocytes	Elliptocytes	Bizarre micropoikilocytosis and fragmented RBCs	Stomatocytes	Target cells, spiculated cells with hemoglobin concentrated in one area of the cells
Anemia	Mild	Mild	Severe	Mild to moderate	Mild to moderate
MCV	Normal	Normal to increased	Markedly decreased	Increased	Increased
MCH	Normal	Normal			
MCHC	Normal to increased	Normal		Decreased	Increased
Osmotic fragility	Increased	Variable	Markedly increased	Increased	Markedly decreased
Autohemolysis test	Increased	Variable	Increased		

REF: H:122–131; L:244–248; M:203–209; T:105–107, 367

54. Males have one X chromosome and one Y chromosome. Females have two X chromosomes. Since G6PD deficiency may be inherited only on the X chromosome, the possible inheritance patterns may be illustrated as follows:

Males: X^+Y or X^-Y

Females: X^+X^+ or X^+X^- or X^-X^- (where X^+ is normal and X^- is G6PD deficiency)

Thus, a hemizygous male will fully express the disorder every time it is inherited. On the other hand, since females have two X chromosomes, full expression of the disorder will occur only when both chromosomes are abnormal. REF: H:135; L:250–251; M:278; T:107

55.

Test	Result	Principle
Hemoglobin	Normal to decreased	Highly sensitive RBCs lyse when exposed to complement
RBC indices	Normal	The abnormality that caused anemia is a membrane defect. Unless the patient has a concurrent iron deficiency, normal-sized cells are formed
Reticulocyte count	Increased	Reticulocytes are produced in response to the anemia
RBC acetylcholinesterase	Decreased	
Leukocyte count	Decreased	The granulocyte membrane is sensitive to the lytic action of complement; thus, destruction of granulocytes results in a lowered WBC count
Leukocyte alkaline phosphatase	Decreased	
Platelet count	Decreased	The platelet membrane is sensitive to the lytic action of complement; thus, destruction of platelets results in a lowered platelet count
Urine hemosiderin	Positive	Chronic hemolysis results in iron lost into the urine. Renal tubular cells catabolize the iron. As the cells are sloughed into the urine, Prussian blue stains will reveal the iron in the urinary sediment
Urine hemoglobin	Positive	Hemoglobin from intravascular hemolysis is cleared by the kidney; thus, the hemoglobin appears in the urine
Indirect hemoglobin	Increased	Bilirubin is a metabolite of excessive breakdown of RBCs during extravascular hemolysis
Plasma hemoglobin	Increased	Free plasma hemoglobin is the result of intravascular hemolysis
Haptoglobin	Decreased	Haptoglobin complexes with plasma hemoglobin and is cleared by the reticuloendothelial system. The "clearing" depletes haptoglobin
Direct antiglobulin test	Negative	PNH is not antibody–mediated
Sugar water test	Positive	The RBCs are hypersensitive to lysis
Acidified serum lysis test/Ham's test	Positive	The RBCs are hypersensitive to lysis
Bone marrow aspiration and biopsy	Erythroid hyperplasia	Production of RBCs is increased in the bone marrow in an effort to compensate for chronic hemolysis

REF: H:185–186; L:263; M:210–212; T:109, 354–355, 367–368

56. A deficiency of complement regulatory proteins results in blood cell membranes that are hypersensitive to the lytic action of complement. REF: H:184; L:262; M:210; T:109

57. A. c
    B. b
    C. b
    D. b
    E. b
    REF: H:196–197; L:234; M:197; T:74–75

58. 50% AS, 50% SS. REF: H:143; L:187; M:156; T:44

59. Levels of hemoglobin S and F, availability of oxygen, presence of other hemoglobinopathies, dehydration, blood viscosity
    REF: H:147; L:197; M:136–137; T:x

60. AA, DD, AS, SC, CC, SS
    REF: H:147–154; L:197–202; M:136–144; T:111, 113

61. A. SS, DD, GG, SD, SG, or DG

    B. SC, SE, GC, GE, DC, DE, SO Arab, DO Arab, or GO Arab

    C. AS, AG, or AD

    D. AA
    REF: H:151; L:193; M:133; T:69–70

62. A. Elevated A_2 and F, small amount of A; thalassemia major
       REF: H:168; L:193, 215; M:133, 153; T:112

    B. Hemoglobins Bart's and Portland; hydrops fetalis syndrome
       REF: H:170; L:193, 216; M:162; T:x

    C. Hemoglobins A and H; hemoglobin H disease
       REF: H:170; L:27, 216; M:161; T:112

    D. Hemoglobins A and A_2; normal
       REF: H:177; L:193; M:38; T:70

63. A. Temporary interruption of hematopoiesis

    B. Increased destruction of RBCs, resulting in a decrease in hemoglobin and hematocrit values

    C. Rigid sickled cells obstruct blood flow through small vessels causing damage and necrosis of tissue.
    REF: H:147; L:197; M:138–139; T:x

64. A. b. REF: H:164; L:186; M:149; T:110

    B. a. REF: H:164; L:186; M:136; T:110

    C. a. REF: H:164; L:186; M:142; T:110

    D. c. REF: H:164; L:186; M:136, 149; T:110

    E. b. REF: H:169; L:186; M:149; T:110

    F. b. REF: H:172; L:224; M:158; T:112

    G. a. REF: H:171; L:186; M:155; T:x

65. A. b. REF: H:170; L:216; M:162; T:112

    B. d. REF: H:170; L:217; M:161; T:112

    C. a. REF: H:171; L:x; M:160; T:x

    D. c. REF: H:171; L:x; M:160; T:111

66. A. A decreased RBC life-span caused by humoral antibody produced against a foreign RBC antigen introduced into the body via transfusion, pregnancy, or organ transplantation. REF: H:194–195; L:267; M:245; T:x

    B. A decreased RBC life-span caused by humoral antibody produced against the person's own RBC antigens. REF: H:194–195; L:267; M:236; T:118

    C. A decreased RBC life-span caused by humoral antibody against a drug or drug complex. REF: H:194–196; L:274; M:242; T:x

    D. Acute intravascular hemolysis occurring within minutes to hours after transfusing incompatible blood. REF: H:196; L:271; M:245; T:x

    E. A shortened RBC life-span in a fetus or newborn due to destruction of the RBCs by antibodies that have crossed the placenta from the mother. REF: H:197; L:270; M:246; T:118–119.

67.

Anemia	RDW	Serum Iron	TIBC	Serum Ferritin	FEP	A₂ Level
Iron deficiency	↑	↓	↑	↓	↑	nl
α-Thalassemia	nl	nl	nl	nl	nl	nl
β-Thalassemia	nl	nl	nl	nl	nl	↑
Hemoglobin E disease	nl	nl	nl	nl	nl	nl
Anemia of chronic disease	nl	↓	↓	↑	↑	nl
Sideroblastic anemia	↑	↑	nl	↑	↓	nl
Lead intoxication	nl	nl	nl	nl	↑	nl

REF: H:180; L:173, 203, 219, 223; M:125, 145, 152, 153, 159; T:101–102, 105, 112–113

68. A. c. REF: H:60; L:246; M:235; T:x

   B. e. REF: H:61; L:245; M:203; T:365–366

   C. a. REF: H:60; L:114; M:88; T:351

   D. f. REF: H:60; L:188; M:132; T:358

   E. d. REF: H:61; L:252; M:216; T:357

   F. b. REF: H:62; L:174; M:117; T:100

69. A. PK deficiency. REF: H:138–139; L:250; M:218; T:71

   B. Immune hemolytic anemia. REF: H:134–141; L:270; M:232; T:109

   C. G6PD deficiency. REF: H:137; L:252; M:216; T:107

   D. Enzyme deficiency not otherwise specified. REF: H:139; L:248; M:212; T:x

   E. Hemoglobin M diseases. REF: H:139; L:82; M:147; T:113

Section One Questions

Select the Best Answer	Answers & References

1. The anticoagulant most often used for cell counting is:
   A. EDTA.
   B. Sodium citrate.
   C. Heparin.
   D. Sodium oxalate.
	A
	H:x
	L:18
	M:100–101
	T:16

2. The anticoagulant most often used for coagulation testing is:
   A. EDTA.
   B. Sodium citrate.
   C. Heparin.
   D. Sodium oxalate.
	B
	H:585
	L:18
	M:407
	T:16–17

3. The main site of hematopoiesis in the fetus from the second to the seventh month is the:
   A. Bone marrow.
   B. Liver.
   C. Kidney.
   D. Yolk sac.
	B
	H:22
	L:47
	M:11
	T:44–45

4. In adulthood, the main site of hematopoiesis is in the:
   A. Axial skeleton.
   B. Distal long bones.
   C. Liver.
   D. Lymph nodes.
	A
	H:22
	L:47
	M:17
	T:45

5. The hematopoietic marrow of the bone is:
   A. A semi-fluid meshwork of stromal cells.
   B. Randomly disbursed throughout the sinusoidal spaces.
   C. Separated from peripheral blood by osteoclasts.
   D. Developed around the bone vasculature.
	D
	H:42
	L:47
	M:x
	T:45

6. The main function of the marrow is to:
   A. Provide mature cells for peripheral circulation.
   B. Synthesize the bone matrix.
   C. Produce collagen, glycoproteins, and proteoglycans.
   D. Provide fat cells for subcutaneous tissue.
	A
	H:44
	L:47
	M:17–18
	T:44

Select the Best Answer	Answers & References

7. The site most often used for bone marrow biopsy and aspiration in adults is the:
  A. Posterior superior iliac crest.
  B. Anterior superior iliac crest.
  C. Sternum.
  D. Spinal processes.
	A
	H:45
	L:366
	M:100
	T:26

8. A bone biopsy is needed when:
  A. The M:E ratio is low.
  B. Anemia is suspected.
  C. Marrow cannot be aspirated.
  D. Fine cellular details are desired.
	C
	H:47
	L:x
	M:102
	T:x

9. Marrow cellularity is determined by comparing:
  A. Granulocytes and their precursors to nucleated RBCs.
  B. Nucleated RBCs to fat cells.
  C. Nucleated hematopoietic cells to granulocytes and their precursors.
  D. Nucleated hematopoietic cells to fat cells.
	D
	H:49
	L:374
	M:102
	T:356

10. The M:E ratio is determined by dividing the number of:
  A. Fat cells by the number of granulocytes and their precursors.
  B. Nucleated RBCs by the number of lymphoid cells.
  C. Granulocytes and their precursors by the number of nucleated RBCs.
  D. Nucleated hematopoietic cells by the number of fat cells.
	C
	H:49
	L:377
	M:101
	T:356

11. The normal M:E ratio in adults is:
  A. 1:1.5 to 1:3.
  B. 2:1 to 4:1.
  C. 1:3 to 1:4.
  D. 3:1 to 4:1.
	B
	H:49
	L:377
	M:101
	T:356

12. The RBC membrane is a(n):
  A. Impermeable lipid membrane surface.
  B. Permeable glycoprotein cytoplasmic membrane.
  C. Semi-permeable lipid bi-layer.
  D. Hypopermeable lipoprotein cytoskeleton.
	C
	H:4
	L:65
	M:28
	T:33

13. The main integral (extrinsic) protein in the RBC is:
  A. Spectrin.
  B. Hemoglobin.
  C. Cholesterol.
  D. Glycophorin.
	D
	H:6
	L:66
	M:28
	T:33

Select the Best Answer	Answers & References
14. The main peripheral (intrinsic) protein in the RBC is: A. Spectrin. B. Hemoglobin. C. Cholesterol. D. Glycophorin.	A H:6 L:65 M:28 T:33
15. The average life-span of a normal RBC is _____ days. A. 7 B. 30 C. 60 D. 120	D H:7 L:58 M:81 T:69
16. Spherocytes and bite cells are evidence of: A. Increased cholesterol. B. Loss of RBC membrane. C. Extravascular hemolysis (catabolism). D. Decreased membrane calcium.	B H:7 L:92 M:x T:91
17. The purpose of the cationic pumps in the RBC are to: A. Actively transport sodium out of the cell and calcium into the cell. B. Actively transport sodium out of the cell and potassium into the cell. C. Passively transport water into the cell and chloride out of the cell. D. Passively transport chloride into the cell and bicarbonate out of the cell.	B H:7 L:66 M:x T:34
18. The carrier protein that delivers iron to the RBC membrane is: A. Protoporphyrin. B. Transferrin. C. Ferritin. D. Hemosiderin.	B H:8 L:78 M:112 T:66
19. If one of the normal enzymatic steps in heme synthesis is blocked or deficient, the resultant disorders are called: A. Porphyrias. B. Thalassemias. C. Methemoglobinemias. D. Hemolytic anemias.	A H:9 L:84 M:126 T:65
20. The globin chains that are usually present *only* during embryonic development are: A. Alpha and beta. B. Zeta and delta. C. Epsilon and zeta. D. Gamma and alpha.	C H:9 L:73 M:38 T:66

Select the Best Answer	Answers & References

21. All normal adult hemoglobins contain a dimer of which chain?
    A. Alpha
    B. Beta
    C. Delta
    D. Gamma
	A
	H:10
	L:73
	M:38
	T:66–67

22. The RBC organic phosphate 2,3-DPG:
    A. Catalyzes porphyrin synthesis.
    B. Controls hemoglobin affinity for oxygen.
    C. Prevents oxidative denaturation of hemoglobin.
    D. Converts methemoglobin to oxyhemoglobin.
	B
	H:12
	L:73
	M:43
	T:62

23. The hemoglobin pigment that *cannot* be converted to oxyhemoglobin is:
    A. Sulfhemoglobin.
    B. Methemoglobin.
    C. Deoxyhemoglobin.
    D. Carboxyhemoglobin.
	A
	H:14
	L:78
	M:45
	T:68

24. Ninety percent of the ATP required for RBC energy is produced by the:
    A. Hexose monophosphate shunt.
    B. Kreb's cycle.
    C. Luebering-Rapoport shunt.
    D. Embden-Meyerhof glycolytic pathway.
	D
	H:15
	L:68
	M:30
	T:71

25. A deficiency in the hexose monophosphate shunt results in:
    A. Schizocytes (schistocytes).
    B. Heinz bodies.
    C. Ferric iron aggregates.
    D. Decreased membrane permeability.
	B
	H:16
	L:67, 100
	M:33
	T:73

26. The majority of senescent RBCs are removed from the body by _____ hemolysis (catabolism).
    A. Denaturing.
    B. In vitro.
    C. Extravascular.
    D. Intravascular.
	C
	H:16
	L:232
	M:197
	T:74

27. The growth factor responsible for regulation of RBC production is:
    A. Interleukin.
    B. Erythropoietin.
    C. Colony-stimulating factor.
    D. Burst forming hormone.
	B
	H:27
	L:59
	M:34
	T:57

Select the Best Answer	Answers & References

28. The RBC precursor that is most plentiful in an aspiration from the normal adult marrow is the:
   A. Rubriblast.
   B. Prorubricyte.
   C. Rubricyte.
   D. Metarubricyte.
	C
	H:29
	L:x
	M:101
	T:356

29. Reticulocytes may be seen in Wright's-stained smears as:
   A. Polychromasia.
   B. Nucleated RBCs.
   C. Spherocytes.
   D. Siderocytes.
	A
	H:30
	L:64
	M:97
	T:60

30. The normal mature RBC is a:
   A. Sphere with a 90 fL diameter.
   B. Sphere with a 7–8 μm diameter.
   C. Bi-concave disc with a 90 fL diameter.
   D. Bi-concave disc with a 6–8 μm diameter.
	D
	H:30
	L:64
	M:27
	T:60

31. Iron found in the bone marrow stores is in the form of:
   A. Ferritin.
   B. Hemosiderin.
   C. Transferrin.
   D. Histiosiderin.
	B
	H:51
	L:237
	M:102
	T:100

32. The packed cell volume is also known as the:
   A. RBC count.
   B. Hemoglobin.
   C. Hematocrit.
   D. Mean cell volume.
	C
	H:57
	L:110
	M:85
	T:347

33. The normal hemoglobin level for people living at high altitudes would be:
   A. The same as people living at sea level.
   B. Higher than people living at sea level.
   C. Lower than people living at sea level.
   D. Unpredictable.
	B
	H:55
	L:127
	M:83
	T:x

34. Approximately _____ percent of RBCs are replaced daily in the adult.
   A. 10.0
   B. 5.0
   C. 2.5
   D. 1.0
	D
	H:55
	L:69
	M:81
	T:60

Select the Best Answer	Answers & References
35. A mechanism in which the body attempts to compensate for anemia is: A. Increased 2,3-DPG. B. Increased WBC production. C. Decreased plasma volume. D. Decreased reticulocyte production.	A H:56 L:73 M:83 T:63
36. The ''rule of three'' suggests that: A. The RBC count is approximately 3 times greater than the hemoglobin value. B. The hematocrit is approximately 3 times greater than the hemoglobin value. C. The WBC count is approximately 3 times greater than the RBC count. D. The hemoglobin value is approximately 3 times greater than the MCV.	B H:57 L:113 M:85 T:x
37. The anemia of a patient whose MCV = 65.1 fL, MCH = 22.2 pg, and MCHC = 295 g/L is termed: A. Normocytic, normochromic. B. Normocytic, hypochromic. C. Microcytic, normochromic. D. Microcytic, hypochromic.	D H:57 L:113–114 M:87 T:76, 87, 91–92
38. A patient whose RBC = 4.01×10^{12}/L, Hb = 125 g/L, and Hct = 0.372 L/L has the following RBC indices: A. MCV = 92.8 fL, MCH = 31.2 pg, MCHC = 336 g/L. B. MCV = 92.8 fL, MCH = 33.6 pg, MCHC = 312 g/L. C. MCV = 107.8 fL, MCH = 32.1 pg, MCHC = 298 g/L. D. MCV = 149.2 fL, MCH = 31.2 pg, MCHC = 336 g/L.	A H:57 L:113–114 M:86–87 T:76
39. The recommended method for hemoglobin measurement is spectrophotometric absorbance reading of: A. Oxyhemoglobin. B. Iron content. C. Cyanmethemoglobin. D. Porphyrin.	C H:59 L:108 M:x T:341
40. A calculated hematocrit is derived from the: A. RBC count and MCHC. B. MCV and hemoglobin. C. MCV and RBC count. D. RBC count and MCH.	C H:59 L:113 M:85 T:311

Select the Best Answer	Answers & References

41. Reticulocytes are:
  A. Nucleated RBCs with cytoplasmic DNA.
  B. Nucleated RBCs with cytoplasmic RNA.
  C. Non-nucleated RBCs with cytoplasmic DNA.
  D. Non-nucleated RBCs with cytoplasmic RNA.
	D
	H:60
	L:64
	M:26
	T:60

42. Body stores of iron are most closely paralleled by serum levels of:
  A. Iron.
  B. Ferritin.
  C. Transferrin.
  D. Vitamin B_{12}.
	B
	H:62
	L:77
	M:x
	T:x

43. Porphyrias are disorders of:
  A. Globin synthesis.
  B. Heme production.
  C. Iron absorption.
  D. Hemoglobin metabolism.
	B
	H:88
	L:84
	M:126
	T:65

44. The hematologic parameter that is most sensitive to macrocytosis is:
  A. Hemoglobin.
  B. Mean cell volume.
  C. Erythrocyte count.
  D. Reticulocyte count.
	B
	H:98
	L:90
	M:87
	T:x

45. When reticulocytes are stained with supravital stains, the substance that stains is:
  A. Hemoglobin.
  B. Hemopexin.
  C. DNA.
  D. RNA.
	D
	H:117
	L:99
	M:26
	T:60

46. Hemoglobin in the ferric (Fe^{3+}) state is called:
  A. Oxyhemoglobin.
  B. Methemoglobin.
  C. Carboxyhemoglobin.
  D. Deoxyhemoglobin.
	B
	H:139
	L:82
	M:44
	T:73

47. The most common adult hemoglobin is:
  A. A.
  B. A_2.
  C. F.
  D. Gower.
	A
	H:144
	L:73
	M:39
	T:67

Select the Best Answer	Answers & References

48. The most common hemoglobin in newborns is:
  A. A.
  B. A_2.
  C. F.
  D. Gower.
	C
	H:144
	L:73
	M:39
	T:66

49. Blood is pipetted to the 0.5 mark of the RBC pipet, and the number of cells counted in the large center primary square on both sides of the hemacytometer equals 2400 RBCs. The RBC count is _____ $\times 10^{12}$/L.
  A. 0.53
  B. 1.20
  C. 2.40
  D. 4.80
	C
	H:525–527
	L:319
	M:x
	T:340–341

50. A reticulocyte count reveals 15 reticulocytes per 1000 RBCs on an 18-year-old white female with iron deficiency. The patient's RBC count is 3.51×10^{12}/L and the hematocrit is 0.271 L/L. The absolute reticulocyte count is _____ $\times 10^9$/L.
  A. 17.5
  B. 25.1
  C. 35.1
  D. 52.6
	D
	H:530
	L:114–117
	M:88–89
	T:352

51. A reticulocyte count reveals 15 reticulocytes per 1000 RBCs on an 18-year-old white female with iron deficiency. The patient's RBC count is 3.51×10^{12}/L and the hematocrit is 0.271 L/L. The uncorrected reticulocyte count is _____%.
  A. 0.5
  B. 1.0
  C. 1.5
  D. 15
	C
	H:530
	L:114–117
	M:88–89
	T:61

52. The iron-laden, nucleated RBC is called a:
  A. Ferricyte.
  B. Ferriblast.
  C. Siderocyte.
  D. Sideroblast.
	D
	H:11
	L:78
	M:98
	T:380

53. The iron-laden, anucleated RBC is called a:
  A. Ferricyte.
  B. Ferriblast.
  C. Siderocyte.
  D. Sideroblast.
	C
	H:11
	L:78
	M:98
	T:380

Select the Best Answer	Answers & References

54. The following RBC histogram is indicative of:
 	
  A. Normal RBCs.
  B. Megaloblastic anemia.
  C. Iron deficiency.
  D. Dimorphic RBC population.
	D
	H:564
	L:505
	M:x
	T:x

Femtoliters

Select the Best Answer	Answers & References

55. A variation in size of RBCs is termed:
  A. Poikilocytosis.
  B. Anisocytosis.
  C. Polychromasia.
  D. Hypochromasia.
	B
	H:66
	L:91
	M:92
	T:87

56. A variation in shape of RBCs is termed:
  A. Poikilocytosis.
  B. Anisocytosis.
  C. Polychromasia.
  D. Hypochromasia.
	A
	H:66
	L:92
	M:92
	T:87

57. Macrocytes can be defined as RBCs with a:
  A. Central pallor greater than one third of the cell.
  B. Mean cell hemoglobin concentration less than 320 g/L.
  C. RBC distribution width greater than 11.
  D. Mean cell volume greater than 98 fL.
	D
	H:66
	L:90
	M:96
	T:x

58. Macrocytosis can be caused by:
  A. Decreased erythropoiesis.
  B. Dietary iron deficiency.
  C. Abnormal DNA production.
  D. Acute hemorrhage.
	C
	H:66
	L:90
	M:96
	T:87

59. Microcytosis can be caused by:
  A. Decreased erythropoiesis.
  B. Dietary iron deficiency.
  C. Impaired DNA synthesis.
  D. Acute hemorrhage.
	B
	H:67
	L:91
	M:97
	T:87

Select the Best Answer	Answers & References

60. Any RBC having an increased central area of pallor is said to have:
  A. Normochromasia.
  B. Polychromasia.
  C. Hypochromasia.
  D. Hyperchromasia.
	C
	H:67
	L:90
	M:97
	T:92

61. A Wright's-stained smear of a patient with an elevated reticulocyte count will show:
  A. Polychromasia.
  B. Rouleaux.
  C. Microcytosis.
  D. Agglutination.
	A
	H:67
	L:99
	M:97
	T:92

62. Cells that are more often artifactual than a true result of a disease process are:
  A. Spherocytes.
  B. Elliptocytes (ovalocytes).
  C. Acanthocytes.
  D. Stomatocytes.
	D
	H:69
	L:94
	M:94
	T:x

63. Cells that occur as a result of a decreased oxygen environment are:
  A. Codocytes (target cells).
  B. Dacryocytes (teardrop cells).
  C. Schizocytes (schistocytes).
  D. Drepanocytes (sickle cells).
	D
	H:69
	L:97
	M:96
	T:91

64. The morphologic difference between acanthocytes and burr cells is evident in the:
  A. Number and length of spicules.
  B. Amount of hemoglobin present.
  C. Shape of the central pallor.
  D. Presence of inclusion bodies.
	A
	H:69–70
	L:93
	M:91
	T:87–88, 90

65. An aid for dealing with RBC agglutination in a laboratory specimen is to:
  A. Replace the plasma with saline.
  B. Warm the specimen.
  C. Mix the specimen immediately after collection.
  D. Remove the plasma.
	B
	H:70
	L:89
	M:99
	T:x

66. An aid for dealing with rouleaux in a laboratory specimen is to:
  A. Replace the plasma with saline.
  B. Warm the specimen.
  C. Mix the specimen immediately after collection.
  D. Remove the plasma.
	A
	H:71
	L:x
	M:99
	T:x

Select the Best Answer	Answers & References

67. A stain used to confirm the presence of precipitated iron in the RBCs is:
    A. Wright's.
    B. New methylene blue N.
    C. Prussian blue.
    D. Cabot's.
	C
	H:71
	L:98
	M:114
	T:380

68. A patient with lead intoxication typically has numerous RBCs with:
    A. Howell-Jolly bodies.
    B. Basophilic stippling.
    C. Pappenheimer bodies.
    D. Heinz bodies.
	B
	H:87
	L:98
	M:98
	T:92

69. Cells that have decreased tolerance to swelling ...d are less deformable than normal are:
    A. Codocytes (target cells).
    B. Discocytes.
    C. Xerocytes.
    D. Spherocytes.
	D
	H:122
	L:92
	M:94
	T:91, 366

70. The RBC with a slit-like central pallor is called a(n):
    A. Elliptocyte.
    B. Stomatocyte.
    C. Erythrocyte.
    D. Spherocyte.
	B
	H:131
	L:94
	M:94
	T:91

71. Heinz bodies are:
    A. Denatured hemoglobin.
    B. Nuclear remnants.
    C. Leftover RNA.
    D. Precipitated iron.
	A
	H:136
	L:207
	M:98
	T:92

72. Heinz bodies can be seen only with _____ stain.
    A. Wright's.
    B. Romanowsky.
    C. Iron.
    D. Supravital.
	D
	H:137
	L:207
	M:98
	T:92

73. Disorders involving any component of hemoglobin synthesis usually result in RBCs that are:
    A. Normocytic, normochromic.
    B. Microcytic, normochromic.
    C. Microcytic, hypochromic.
    D. Macrocytic, hyperchromic.
	C
	H:77
	L:113–114
	M:119
	T:87, 92

Select the Best Answer	Answers & References

74. In the body, iron primarily acts as a(n):
    A. Oxygen transporter.
    B. Energy enhancer.
    C. Bacteriocidal agent.
    D. Stimulus for porphyrin synthesis.
	A
	H:77
	L:172
	M:82
	T:62

75. The majority of iron in the body is found in the:
    A. Liver.
    B. Bone marrow.
    C. Spleen.
    D. RBCs.
	D
	H:78
	L:77
	M:110
	T:99

76. Eating foods high in vitamin C along with iron-rich foods will cause iron absorption to be:
    A. Unchanged.
    B. Increased.
    C. Decreased.
    D. Variable.
	B
	H:79
	L:175
	M:111
	T:99

77. Pappenheimer bodies are also known as:
    A. Prussian bodies.
    B. Basophilic stippling.
    C. Siderotic granules.
    D. Porphyrias.
	C
	H:79
	L:98
	M:98
	T:93

78. The most common cause of iron deficiency in American women of childbearing years is:
    A. Gastrointestinal bleeding.
    B. Menstrual bleeding.
    C. Dietary insufficiency.
    D. Urinary excretion.
	B
	H:84
	L:175
	M:115
	T:99

79. The most common cause of iron deficiency in adult men is:
    A. Dietary insufficiency.
    B. Repeated blood donations.
    C. Malabsorption syndromes.
    D. Gastrointestinal bleeding.
	D
	H:84
	L:175
	M:116
	T:99

80. During treatment for iron deficiency anemia, recovery is first seen in the peripheral blood as:
    A. A dual population of RBCs.
    B. Return of hemoglobin levels to normal.
    C. Macrocytic, normochromic reversal.
    D. Increased siderocytes.
	A
	H:85
	L:177
	M:x
	T:x

Select the Best Answer	Answers & References

81. Hemosiderosis is:
  A. An autosomal recessive disease characterized by elevated iron absorption.
  B. An aplastic anemia characterized by ringed sideroblasts.
  C. A disorder in which RBC precursors store iron in ribosomes.
  D. The deposition of excess iron in macrophages of tissues such as the liver and spleen.
	D
	H:85
	L:99
	M:115
	T:x

82. In pernicious anemia, the large NRBC with a webby chromatin pattern is a:
  A. Rubriblast.
  B. Macroblast.
  C. Megaloblast.
  D. Megakaryoblast.
	C
	H:92
	L:158
	M:x
	T:x

83. A group of drugs that commonly interferes with normal DNA metabolism is:
  A. Antibiotics.
  B. Chemotherapeutics.
  C. Antiarrhythmics.
  D. Diuretics.
	B
	H:93
	L:90
	M:180
	T:x

84. The protein needed for vitamin B_{12} to be absorbed from food into the intestinal mucosa is:
  A. Transcobalamin II.
  B. Pteroylglutamine.
  C. Albumin.
  D. Intrinsic factor.
	D
	H:94
	L:156
	M:178
	T:103

85. The primary cause of folic acid deficiency is:
  A. Malabsorption.
  B. Increased utilization.
  C. Increased loss.
  D. Decreased dietary intake.
	D
	H:95
	L:156
	M:172
	T:103

86. The primary cause of vitamin B_{12} deficiency is:
  A. Malabsorption.
  B. Increased utilization.
  C. Increased loss.
  D. Decreased dietary intake.
	A
	H:97
	L:161
	M:177
	T:104

87. Evidence indicates that the cause of pernicious anemia is:
  A. Old age.
  B. Overexposure to certain drugs.
  C. Autoantibodies to parietal cells.
  D. Liver dysfunction.
	C
	H:97
	L:160
	M:177
	T:104

Select the Best Answer	Answers & References

88. The clinical manifestation that distinguishes pernicious anemia from folic acid deficiency is:
  A. Neurologic abnormality.
  B. Shortness of breath.
  C. Fatigue.
  D. Slight jaundice.
	A
	H:98
	L:159
	M:168
	T:x

89. When the maturation rates of nuclear and cytoplasmic development of hematopoietic cells differ, it is called:
  A. Asynchrony.
  B. Karyorrhexis.
  C. Pyknosis.
  D. Hyperplasia.
	C
	H:100
	L:x
	M:169
	T:x

90. In megaloblastic anemias, the M:E ratio of the bone marrow is often:
  A. Normal.
  B. Decreased.
  C. Increased.
  D. Variable.
	B
	H:100
	L:x
	M:169
	T:x

91. A major cause of non-megaloblastic macrocytosis is:
  A. Iron deficiency.
  B. Alcoholism.
  C. Folic acid deficiency.
  D. Pernicous anemia.
	B
	H:101
	L:164
	M:181
	T:x

92. A chemistry test that is often elevated in patients with megaloblastic anemia is:
  A. Creatine phosphokinase.
  B. Serum protein.
  C. Lactic dehydrogenase.
  D. Amylase.
	C
	H:103
	L:160
	M:170
	T:104

93. Following correct diagnosis and treatment of a megaloblastic anemia, the patient's complete blood count (CBC) returns to normal in approximately:
  A. 3–4 days.
  B. 1–2 weeks.
  C. 4–6 weeks.
  D. 4–6 months.
	C
	H:104
	L:163
	M:x
	T:x

94. Aplastic anemia manifests as a decreased production of:
  A. Megakaryocytic precursors.
  B. Myeloid precursors.
  C. Erythroid precursors.
  D. All hematopoietic precursors.
	D
	H:108
	L:138
	M:185
	T:97–98

Select the Best Answer	Answers & References

95. One of the more common causes of aplastic anemia is:
  A. Exposure to benzene compounds.
  B. Exposure to ionizing radiation.
  C. Overwhelming infections.
  D. Genetic inheritance.
	A
	H:109
	L:139
	M:188
	T:98

96. A drug that frequently causes aplastic anemia is:
  A. Sulfonamide.
  B. Streptomycin.
  C. Chloramphenicol.
  D. Aspirin.
	C
	H:109
	L:139
	M:187
	T:98

97. An infectious state that is occasionally associated with bone marrow suppression is:
  A. Strep throat.
  B. Hepatitis.
  C. Chicken pox.
  D. Pneumococcal pneumonia.
	B
	H:110
	L:338
	M:188
	T:98

98. Clinical manifestations of aplastic anemia are the result of:
  A. Splenomegaly.
  B. Lymphadenopathy.
  C. Pancytopenia.
  D. Malabsorption.
	C
	H:111
	L:140
	M:185
	T:98

99. Peripheral blood cell morphology in aplastic anemia is most often:
  A. Normocytic, normochromic.
  B. Microcytic, hypochromic.
  C. Macrocytic, normochromic.
  D. Microcytic, hyperchromic.
	A
	H:111
	L:140
	M:189
	T:x

100. The reticulocyte count of a patient with aplastic anemia is usually:
  A. Normal.
  B. Increased.
  C. Decreased.
  D. Variable.
	C
	H:111
	L:141
	M:180
	T:x

101. In aplastic anemia, an abnormality that may be noted in the WBC differential is:
  A. Relative lymphocytosis.
  B. Absolute lymphocytosis.
  C. Relative neutrophilia.
  D. Absolute neutrophilia.
	A
	H:111
	L:x
	M:189
	T:x

Select the Best Answer	Answers & References
102. In aplastic anemia, a bone marrow biopsy commonly reveals a marrow that is: A. Normocellular. B. Hypocellular. C. Hypercellular. D. Extracellular.	B H:111 L:141 M:189 T:x
103. If left untreated, most patients with aplastic anemia will: A. Spontaneously recover. B. Develop leukemia. C. Gradually improve. D. Die.	D H:111 L:141 M:190 T:x
104. For children and young adults with severe aplastic anemia, the preferred treatment is: A. Supportive therapy. B. Immunosuppressive therapy. C. Antibiotics. D. Bone marrow transplantation.	D H:111 L:141 M:190 T:98
105. Anemia of chronic disease (inflammation) is usually a: A. Mild microcytic, hypochromic anemia. B. Severe macrocytic, normochromic anemia. C. Severe microcytic, hyperchromic anemia. D. Mild normocytic, normochromic anemia.	D H:225 L:178 M:125 T:102
106. Anemia of chronic disease (inflammation) may be confused initially with iron deficiency anemia because both disorders exhibit: A. Low serum iron levels. B. Low iron stores in reticuloendothelial cells. C. Elevated total iron binding capacities. D. Elevated reticulocyte counts.	A H:225 L:173 M:125 T:101–102
107. In inflammation, the erythrocyte sedimentation rate is often: A. Elevated. B. Decreased. C. Normal. D. Variable.	A H:225 L:120 M:x T:353
108. The primary cause of anemia of chronic renal disease is: A. Hemolysis resulting from capillary thrombosis. B. Decreased erythropoietin production. C. Suppression of erythropoiesis by uremic toxins. D. Blood lost in the urine.	B H:233 L:147 M:35 T:58

Select the Best Answer	Answers & References

109. Round macrocytes, acanthocytes, and codocytes (target cells) are typical in anemia associated with:
  A. Endocrine disease.
  B. Renal disease.
  C. Liver disease.
  D. Infection.
	C
	H:234
	L:90,93–94
	M:189
	T:88–91

110. During and immediately following alcohol abuse, the MCV will be:
  A. Elevated.
  B. Decreased.
  C. Normal.
  D. Variable.
	A
	H:235
	L:91
	M:182–183
	T:x

111. A decreased haptoglobin level, hemoglobinemia, and hemoglobinuria are indicative of ＿＿ hemolysis (catabolism).
  A. No.
  B. Intravascular.
  C. Extravascular.
  D. Anoxic.
	B
	H:18
	L:234
	M:197
	T:74–75

112. Osmotic fragility tests on patients with a high number of spherocytes in the peripheral blood will be:
  A. Normal.
  B. Increased.
  C. Decreased.
  D. Variable.
	B
	H:61
	L:245
	M:205
	T:367

113. If codocytes (target cells) are seen on the peripheral blood smear, the osmotic fragility will be:
  A. Normal.
  B. Increased.
  C. Decreased.
  D. Variable.
	C
	H:68
	L:245
	M:205
	T:367

114. When RBCs from a patient with an intracorpuscular RBC defect are transfused into a healthy individual, the life-span of the RBCs will be:
  A. Less than normal.
  B. Normal.
  C. Greater than normal.
  D. Variable.
	A
	H:116
	L:x
	M:201
	T:x

Select the Best Answer	Answers & References

115. When RBCs from a healthy donor are transfused into a patient with an extracorpuscular RBC defect, the life-span of the donor cells will be:
  A. Less than normal.
  B. Normal.
  C. Greater than normal.
  D. Variable.
	A
	H:116
	L:x
	M:201
	T:x

116. Hemoglobinemia, hemoglobinuria, and hemosiderinuria are good indicators of:
  A. Ineffective erythropoiesis.
  B. Intravascular hemolysis (catabolism).
  C. Extravascular hemolysis (catabolism).
  D. Intracorpuscular defects.
	B
	H:116
	L:234
	M:197
	T:74−75

117. Cells that have a decreased osmotic fragility and are less deformable than normal are:
  A. Stomatocytes.
  B. Spherocytes.
  C. Xerocytes.
  D. Hydrocytes.
	C
	H:131
	L:248
	M:209
	T:107

118. Hereditary spherocytosis is considered a disorder of the:
  A. Nucleus.
  B. Cytoplasm.
  C. Membrane.
  D. Hemoglobin.
	C
	H:122
	L:92
	M:202
	T:104−105

119. A common treatment for hereditary spherocytosis is:
  A. Splenectomy.
  B. Transfusion therapy.
  C. Spectrin replacement.
  D. Prophylactic penicillin.
	A
	H:124
	L:246
	M:206
	T:106

120. The osmotic fragility in most patients with hereditary elliptocytosis is:
  A. Increased.
  B. Normal.
  C. Decreased.
  D. Variable.
	B
	H:128--129
	L:247
	M:207
	T:x

121. The disorder in which RBCs exhibit thermal instability is hereditary:
  A. Spherocytosis.
  B. Elliptocytosis.
  C. Xerocytosis.
  D. Pyropoikilocytosis.
	D
	H:130
	L:96
	M:209
	T:x

Select the Best Answer	Answers & References

122. The most commonly encountered anemia in the congenital non-spherocytic hemolytic anemias is caused by a deficiency of:
   A. Pyruvate kinase.
   B. Methemoglobin reductase.
   C. Glucose-6-phosphate dehydrogenase.
   D. Glucose phosphate isomerase.
	C
	H:134
	L:250
	M:213
	T:x

123. G6PD is found in the:
   A. Embden-Meyerhof pathway.
   B. Hexose monophosphate shunt.
   C. Luebering-Rapoport pathway.
   D. Methemoglobin reductase pathway.
	B
	H:135
	L:68
	M:32,213
	T:72

124. The hemolytic episodes in G6PD deficient patients are self-limiting because:
   A. The body cannot function with a loss of over 10% of the RBCs.
   B. The antibody causing the hemolysis is depleted.
   C. Young RBCs have nearly normal G6PD levels.
   D. Males have only one X chromosome.
	C
	H:137
	L:257–258
	M:214
	T:x

125. An osmotic fragility performed on fresh blood from a patient with PK deficiency will be:
   A. Normal.
   B. Variable.
   C. Decreased.
   D. Increased.
	A
	H:138
	L:x
	M:218
	T:x

126. Favism may be associated with:
   A. G6PD deficiency.
   B. PK deficiency.
   C. Methemoglobin reductase deficiency.
   D. Non-glycolytic enzyme deficiency.
	A
	H:136
	L:252
	M:214
	T:107

127. PNH is a disorder that is:
   A. Sex-linked recessive.
   B. Autosomal dominant.
   C. Autosomal recessive.
   D. Acquired.
	D
	H:184
	L:262
	M:210
	T:109

128. The classic presentation of a patient with PNH includes:
   A. Hemoglobin in the first morning urine.
   B. Manifestation soon after birth.
   C. Chronic leukocytosis.
   D. Megaloblastic anemia.
	A
	H:185
	L:x
	M:210
	T:109

Select the Best Answer	Answers & References
129. A disorder that may be confused with PNH because both produce positive acidified serum lysis (Ham's) result is: A. Chronic myelogenous leukemia. B. HEMPAS (CDA-II). C. Sideroblastic anemia. D. Iron deficiency anemia.	B H:185, 187 L:264 M:212 T:x
130. Polychromasia may be seen on the Wright's-stained smear of a patient with PNH due to an elevation of: A. Leukocyte alkaline phosphatase. B. Granulocytes. C. RBCs. D. Reticulocytes.	D H:185–186 L:64 M:26, 210 T:92
131. The RBC enzyme whose level corresponds to the acuity of PNH is: A. Alkaline phosphatase. B. Properdin. C. Acetylcholinesterase. D. C5 convertase.	C H:186 L:263 M:210 T:x
132. A screening test for PNH is the: A. Sugar water test. B. Plasma hemoglobin. C. Acidified serum lysis (Ham's) test. D. Urinalysis.	A H:186 L:263 M:211 T:77
133. The confirmatory test for PNH is the: A. Sugar water test. B. Plasma hemoglobin. C. Acidified serum lysis (Ham's) test. D. Urinalysis.	C H:186 L:263 M:211 T:77
134. Fresh normal serum is required for the acidified serum lysis (Ham's) test to ensure the presence of: A. Acetylcholinesterase. B. Complement. C. Acid. D. Antibodies.	B H:186–187 L:x M:211 T:355
135. A valuable test for evaluating suspected hemoglobinopathies is: A. Bone marrow smear and biopsy. B. Hemoglobin electrophoresis. C. Reticulocyte count. D. Haptoglobin assay.	B H:60 L:188 M:132 T:358

Select the Best Answer	Answers & References

136. Hemoglobinopathy may be defined as:
  A. The inheritance of two alpha and two beta chains.
  B. The production of an abnormal hemoglobin.
  C. The presence of high levels of hemoglobin A_1 in adults.
  D. A membrane disorder that reduces RBC oxygen-carrying ability.
	B
	H:143
	L:186
	M:131
	T:68

137. The hemoglobin of sickle cell disease may be designated as:
  A. $\alpha_2\beta_2$.
  B. $\alpha_2\beta_2^{6glu \rightarrow lys}$.
  C. $\alpha_2^{G\ Phil}\beta_2^A$.
  D. $\alpha_2\beta_2^{6glu \rightarrow val}$.
	D
	H:144
	L:186
	M:38, 134
	T:x

138. When the bone marrow temporarily ceases to produce cells in a sickle cell patient, a(n) _____ crisis has occurred.
  A. Aplastic
  B. Hemolytic
  C. Vaso-occlusive
  D. Painful
	A
	H:147
	L:197
	M:138
	T:x

139. The most severe anemia results from which of the following hemoglobinopathies?
  A. SC
  B. SS
  C. AS
  D. SD
	B
	H:147
	L:198
	M:136
	T:110–111

140. The presence of HbF causes the severity of sickling in sickle cell disease to:
  A. Remain the same.
  B. Decrease.
  C. Increase.
  D. Return to normal.
	B
	H:147
	L:x
	M:136
	T:x

141. Hemoglobins that denature and precipitate within RBCs as Heinz bodies are:
  A. Methemoglobinemias.
  B. Thalassemias.
  C. Unstable hemoglobins.
  D. Hemoglobin M.
	C
	H:156
	L:100
	M:145
	T:114

142. The majority of hemoglobinopathies are caused by:
  A. Iron in the reduced state.
  B. Single amino acid substitutions in the globin chain.
  C. Failure to synthesize adequate quantities of globin chains.
  D. Decreased production of porphyrin rings.
	B
	H:143
	L:186
	M:131
	T:110

Select the Best Answer	Answers & References

143. The structural formula $\alpha_2\beta_2^{6glu\rightarrow val}$ indicates that:
   A. Valine has been substituted for glutamic acid in the sixth position.
   B. Glutamic acid has been substituted for valine in the sixth position.
   C. Normal hemoglobin will be produced.
   D. A coding error has occurred in the alpha chain.
	A
	 H:145
	 L:186–187
	 M:142
	 T:x

144. The sickle cell trait patient (AS):
   A. Will never have a sickling crisis.
   B. Usually has sickled cells on the peripheral blood smear.
   C. Is normally asymptomatic.
   D. Shows a predominance of hemoglobin S.
	C
	 H:147
	 L:199
	 M:141
	 T:119

145. The hemoglobin combination SD creates a laboratory problem because:
   A. There are no normal alpha chains produced.
   B. Hemoglobin F is reduced in the newborn.
   C. Hemoglobin D does not sickle.
   D. Hemoglobin D travels with S on alkaline electrophoresis.
	D
	 H:156
	 L:193
	 M:133
	 T:70

146. Methemoglobinemia results in cyanosis and hypoxia because:
   A. Heinz bodies cause the spleen to sequester the RBCs.
   B. Iron is in the oxidized ferric (Fe^{3+}) form.
   C. Iron is in the reduced ferrous (Fe^{2+}) form.
   D. The switchover from gamma to beta chains is prevented.
	B
	 H:156
	 L:82
	 M:147
	 T:68, 113

147. A common characteristic of many hemoglobinopathies is:
   A. Heinz bodies.
   B. Drepanocytes (sickle cells).
   C. Codocytes (target cells).
   D. Spherocytes.
	C
	 H:150–155
	 L:188
	 M:140–144
	 T:91

148. A specimen from a 30-year-old Cambodian immigrant was referred to the laboratory for workup of microcytic, hypochromic RBCs without anemia. A probable cause is inheritance of:
   A. Beta-thalassemia major.
   B. HbSS.
   C. HbSC.
   D. HbEE.
	D
	 H:154
	 L:x
	 M:144
	 T:113

149. Polycythemia or anemia may be the result of:
   A. Hemoglobin variants with altered oxygen affinity.
   B. Hemoglobin S/beta-thalassemia combination.
   C. Sickle cell disease.
   D. Hemoglobin SC disease.
	A
	 H:156
	 L:188
	 M:138
	 T:x

Select the Best Answer	Answers & References
150. The thalassemia syndromes are the result of:	C
A. Amino acid substitutions in the globin chains.	H:164
B. Ineffective iron utilization.	L:212
C. Defective production of globin chains.	M:149
D. Overproduction of protoporphyrin.	T:111
151. Hemoglobin Bart's is designated as:	A
A. γ_4.	H:166
B. $\alpha_2\gamma_2$.	L:204
C. β_4.	M:160
D. $\alpha_2\beta_2$.	T:x
152. Hemoglobin H is designated as:	C
A. γ_4.	H:166
B. $\alpha_2\gamma_2$.	L:204
C. β_4.	M:159
D. $\alpha_2\beta_2$.	T:112
153. Beta-thalassemia is manifested:	C
A. In utero.	H:167
B. At birth.	L:220
C. Several months after birth.	M:151
D. In adulthood.	T:112
154. Beta-thalassemia is characterized by an increase in hemoglobins:	B
A. A and A_2.	H:167
B. A_2 and F.	L:221
C. F and Gower 1.	M:150
D. Bart's and H.	T:112
155. The β^0-thalassemia gene results in:	A
A. Zero production of beta globin chains.	H:167
B. Decreased production of beta globin chains.	L:221
C. Increased production of beta globin chains.	M:149
D. Normal production of abnormal beta globin chains.	T:x
156. The β^+-thalassemia gene results in:	B
A. Zero production of beta globin chains.	H:167
B. Decreased production of beta globin chains.	L:x
C. Increased production of beta globin chains.	M:149
D. Normal production of abnormal beta globin chains.	T:x

Select the Best Answer	Answers & References
157. Alpha-thalassemia is usually manifested: 　A. In utero. 　B. At birth. 　C. Several months after birth. 　D. In adulthood.	B H:169 L:217 M:159 T:x
158. Alpha-thalassemia are characterized by increases in hemoglobins: 　A. A and A_2. 　B. A_2 and F. 　C. F and Gower 1. 　D. Bart's and H.	D H:169–170 L:217–218 M:159 T:112
159. After incubation with brilliant cresyl blue, RBCs containing hemoglobin H will: 　A. Have golfball-like inclusions. 　B. Have reticulocyte-like threads. 　C. Hemolyze. 　D. Form sickled cells.	A H:170–171 L:217 M:x T:x
160. The characteristic that allows hemoglobin F to be studied is its: 　A. Resistance to acid and alkali denaturation. 　B. Electrophoretic movement on citrate agar (pH 6.0). 　C. Presence in all normal RBCs. 　D. Production early in life.	A H:172, 178 L:194 M:132 T:69
161. The thalassemia syndromes are morphologically described as: 　A. Microcytic, hypochromic. 　B. Normocytic, normochromic. 　C. Macrocytic, normochromic. 　D. Megaloblastic, hyperchromic.	A H:176 L:214 M:152 T:112
162. In general, thalassemias are characterized by a(n): 　A. Normal RBC count and elevated hemoglobin. 　B. Decreased RBC count and decreased hemoglobin. 　C. Decreased RBC count and normal hemoglobin. 　D. Elevated RBC count and decreased hemoglobin.	D H:176 L:214 M:x T:x
163. The Kleihauer-Betke acid elution test demonstrates hemoglobin: 　A. A. 　B. A_2. 　C. C. 　D. F.	D H:172 L:194, 210 M:133 T:69

Select the Best Answer	Answers & References

Use for questions 164–166. Given the following laboratory results, identify the hemoglobinopathy for each patient.

Patient	A$_2$ by Column Chromatography	Acid Elution for Hb F	Sickle Solubility Test
Patient A	2.0%	Even distribution	Negative
Patient B	1.0%	Negative	Positive
Patient C	1.5%	Negative	Negative

164. Using the information above, the interpretation for patient A is:

   A. AS.

   B. Hereditary persistence of fetal hemoglobin.

   C. SS.

   D. CD or CG.

> B
> H:537–540
> L:191–194, 225–228
> M:132–134, 141
> T:67, 69–70, 361–362

165. Using the information above, the interpretation for patient B is:

   A. AS.

   B. Hereditary persistence of fetal hemoglobin.

   C. SS.

   D. CD or CG.

> A
> H:537–540
> L:191–194, 225–228
> M:132–134, 141
> T:70, 361–362

166. Using the information above, the interpretation for patient C is:

   A. AS.

   B. Hereditary persistence of fetal hemoglobin.

   C. SS.

   D. CD or CG.

> D
> H:537–540
> L:191–194, 225–228
> M:132–134, 141
> T:70, 361–362

167. A positive direct antiglobulin test is one indication of:

   A. Autoimmune hemolytic anemia.

   B. Iron deficiency anemia.

   C. Pernicious anemia.

   D. Hereditary spherocytosis.

> A
> H:60
> L:246
> M:235
> T:118

168. A delayed hemolytic transfusion reaction occurs within _____ post-transfusion:

   A. 6–12 hours

   B. 12–24 hours

   C. 1–2 days

   D. 2–14 days

> D
> H:197
> L:271
> M:245
> T:x

Select the Best Answer	Answers & References

169. The system most commonly associated with immediate hemolytic transfusion reactions is:
   A. Rh.
   B. ABO.
   C. Kidd.
   D. Duffy.
	B
	H:196
	L:271
	M:x
	T:x

170. The fetomaternal incompatibility most commonly associated with HDN is:
   A. Rh.
   B. ABO.
   C. Kidd.
   D. Lewis.
	B
	H:198
	L:x
	M:x
	T:119

171. In hemolytic disease of the newborn, if intervention therapy is necessary and the fetus is too premature for delivery, the therapy of choice is:
   A. Abortion.
   B. Maternal plasmapheresis.
   C. Intrauterine transfusion.
   D. Phototherapy.
	C
	H:200
	L:270
	M:248
	T:x

172. The specificity of the antibody most commonly found in warm autoimmune hemolytic anemia is:
   A. Anti-e.
   B. Anti-I.
   C. Broad-based anti-ABO.
   D. Broad-based anti-Rh.
	D
	H:203
	L:273
	M:x
	T:x

173. The antibody screen of a patient with warm autoimmune hemolytic anemia (AIHA) will reveal positive results only in the phase associated with:
   A. Immediate spin.
   B. Room temperature incubation.
   C. 37°C incubation.
   D. Anti-human globulin.
	D
	H:203
	L:x
	M:238
	T:x

174. Cold antibodies are usually:
   A. IgA.
   B. IgE.
   C. IgG.
   D. IgM.
	D
	H:204
	L:272
	M:239
	T:118

Select the Best Answer	Answers & References

175. The most common antibody specificity in cold AIHA is:
    A. Anti-e.
    B. Anti-i.
    C. Anti-I.
    D. Anti-P.
	C
	H:204
	L:273
	M:239
	T:x

176. The antibody specificity in paroxysmal cold hemoglobinuria is:
    A. Anti-e.
    B. Anti-I.
    C. Anti-i.
    D. Anti-P.
	D
	H:206
	L:272
	M:241
	T:x

177. The Donath-Landsteiner antibody is associated with:
    A. Paroxysmal cold hemoglobinuria.
    B. Paroxysmal nocturnal hemoglobinuria.
    C. Infectious mononucleosis.
    D. *Mycoplasma pneumoniae.*
	A
	H:206
	L:274
	M:241
	T:356

178. The most common protozoal infestation that results in anemia is:
    A. *Babesia.*
    B. *Plasmodium.*
    C. *Bartonella.*
    D. *Clostridium.*
	B
	H:210–211
	L:262
	M:136, 222
	T:93

179. A common finding in the peripheral blood of patients with intravascular hemolysis due to mechanical trauma is:
    A. Parasites.
    B. Antibodies.
    C. Codocytes (target cells).
    D. Schizocytes (schistocytes).
	D
	H:217
	L:94
	M:94
	T:91

Section Two

—— ❦ ——

LEUKOCYTES

Objectives for Leukocyte Section

---- ❦ ----

After studying the referenced material for each white blood cells (WBCs) chapter outline, completing the worksheet, and taking the section test, the student will be able to:

1 List the developmental changes that occur in the granulocytic, monocytic, and lymphocytic cell lines

2 Differentiate between the maturation stages of WBCs

3 Explain the functions of neutrophils, eosinophils, basophils, monocytes, lymphocytes, and plasma cells

4 Evaluate WBC counts and differentials and apply appropriate descriptive terminology

5 Identify common causes of quantitative and qualitative disorders of leukocytes

6 Name ways to eliminate artifacts that frequently occur when preparing blood smears for morphologic evaluation

7 Calculate manual WBC counts, absolute differential counts, and WBC corrections for nucleated RBCs

8 Describe nuclear and cytoplasmic changes that occur in WBCs as a result of disease states or inheritance

9 Relate the interaction of lymphocyte subsets and monocytes in immune reactions

10 Interpret laboratory data and give a likely diagnosis

11 Select appropriate cytochemical stains to use in differentiating leukemias

12 Classify acute leukemias and myelodysplastic syndromes according to common nomenclature and the French-American-British (FAB) classification

13 Classify acute lymphocytic leukemias according to immunologic markers

14 Distinguish between the chronic myeloproliferative disorders (polycythemia vera, myeloid metaplasia, essential thrombocythemia, chronic myelocytic leukemia, and juvenile chronic myelocytic leukemia)

15 Distinguish between the chronic lymphoproliferative disorders (chronic lymphocytic leukemia, prolymphocytic leukemia, and hairy cell leukemia)

16 Discuss the side effects of chemotherapy for leukemia

17 Label the anatomy of the lymph node

18 Compare and contrast Hodgkin's disease and non-Hodgkin's lymphoma

19 Recognize typical abnormal laboratory results that indicate acquired immune deficiency syndrome (AIDS)

20 Point out differences in the plasma cell disorders (multiple myeloma, Waldenström's macroglobulinemia, plasma cell leukemia, and heavy chain disease)

21 State the purpose of the following laboratory tests:

Acid phosphatase stain
B-cell markers
Bence-Jones protein
Blood viscosity
Cerebrospinal fluid examination
Common acute lymphocytic leukemia
    antigen
Cryoglobulins
Cytogenetics studies
Cytomegalovirus titer
Cytoplasmic immunoglobulin
Direct basophil count
Direct eosinophil count
Epstein-Barr virus titer
Erythropoietin level
Esterase stains
Helper T lymphocyte count
Heterophile antibodies
HIV antibodies

Immunoelectrophoresis
Lupus erythematosus (LE) preparation
Leukocyte alkaline phosphatase stain
Lymph node biopsy
Muramidase
Myeloperoxidase stain
Periodic acid-Schiff stain
RBC mass
Serum protein electrophoresis
Sudan black B stain
T-cell markers
Tartrate-resistant acid phosphatase
Terminal deoxynucleotidyl transferase
Thorn test
Toluidine blue stain
WBC correction for nucleated RBCs
WBC count
WBC differential
WBC histogram

Chapter 8

Leukopoiesis: The Granulocytes

I. Developmental changes: As the cell matures, the nuclear volume decreases, the chromatin becomes coarser as the nucleolus disappears, primary granules appear and then disappear as secondary granules form, the cytoplasm changes from blue to pinkish-red, and the cell size decreases.

A. Myeloblast: Earliest recognizable cell in the granulocytic series. The diameter is 15 to 20 micrometers with the nucleus comprising the majority of the cell. Nucleoli are clearly visible within an open network of chromatin. The cytoplasm is medium-blue.

B. Promyelocyte: The diameter is 15 to 20 micrometers. Primary (non-specific) granules distinguish this cell from the myeloblast. Slight nuclear clumping occurs near the nucleoli and the cytoplasm remains medium-blue.

C. Myelocyte: The diameter is 12 to 18 micrometers. Primary granules are no longer formed, allowing secondary (specific) granules to predominate. The nucleus is round and increasingly coarse. The cytoplasm takes on a slightly pink hue.

D. Metamyelocyte: The diameter is 10 to 15 micrometers. The indented nucleus and absence of nucleoli distinguish this cell from its precursor. The cytoplasm has a pinkish tinge and numerous secondary granules.

E. Band neutrophil: The diameter is 9 to 15 micrometers. The condensed nucleus is indented more than halfway but has not segmented.

F. Segmented neutrophil (polymorphonuclear leukocyte): The diameter is 9 to 15 micrometers. The nucleus usually has two to five lobes with a narrow filament connecting the segments. The cytoplasm is salmon-colored with neutrophilic granules.

G. Tissue neutrophil: Fixed tissue cells with neutrophilic granules.

H. Eosinophil: Large reddish-orange granules fill the cytoplasm. The nucleus is often bi-lobed or band-shaped.

I. Tissue eosinophil: Fixed tissue variants of the motile eosinophil.

J. Basophil: Large blackish-blue granules in the cytoplasm often obscure the nucleus.

K. Tissue basophil (mast cell): Fixed tissue cells with abundant dark-staining granules.

II. Kinetics: Under the direction of colony-stimulating factors, the cells mature within the bone marrow and then cross into the peripheral blood through the sinusoidal spaces. In the blood, the cells are a part of the circulating pool or the marginating pool. Within hours, the cells enter the tissues by diapedesis where they are short-lived. Chemotactic factors attract granulocytes to the site of infection or injury where phagocytosis of foreign substances occurs.

III. Function

A. Neutrophils: Phagocytosis of bacteria and other foreign organisms protects the body from infection. Opsonins enhance phagocytosis.

B. Eosinophils: Limiting allergic reactions prevents generalized allergies, and digestion of parasites helps protect the body from infestation.

C. Basophils: Immediate hypersensitivity reactions are enhanced by histamine released from basophil granules. Similar involvement in delayed hypersensitivity has been noted.

IV. Quantitative disorders of granulocytes

A. Neutrophilia

   1. Cause.
      a. Increased production and release from the bone marrow due to such disorders as bacterial infection, acute injury, leukemia, or cellular necrosis. The increased number is often accompanied by a "shift to the left" indicating early release of immature granulocytes from the bone marrow.
      b. Maldistribution between the marginating and circulating pools due to such disorders as physical or emotional stress.
   2. Laboratory evaluation: The absolute neutrophil count is greater than $6.5 \times 10^9/L$.
 B. Neutropenia
   1. Cause.
      a. Decreased production by the bone marrow due to such disorders as Fanconi's anemia, aplastic anemia, toxic injury, or pernicious anemia
      b. Impaired release from the bone marrow due to such disorders as cyclic neutropenia or acquired agranulocytosis
      c. Increased destruction in the peripheral circulation due to such disorders as splenomegaly, isoimmune neonatal neutropenia, or overwhelming infections
      d. Maldistribution between the marginating and circulating pools due to such disorders as viremia, dialysis, or prolonged bed rest
   2. Laboratory evaluation: The absolute neutrophil count is less than $1.5 \times 10^9/L$.

V. Quantitative disorders of eosinophils
 A. Eosinophilia
   1. Cause: Increased production by the bone marrow due to such disorders as allergies, parasitic infestations, certain malignancies, or inheritance.
   2. Laboratory evaluation: The direct eosinophil count is greater than $0.7 \times 10^9/L$.
 B. Eosinopenia
   1. Cause: Decreased production by the bone marrow may be due to conditions similar to those causing neutropenia. In addition, adrenocorticotrophic hormone (ACTH) administration results in a decreased count in normal individuals.
   2. Laboratory evaluation: The direct eosinophil count is less than $0.05 \times 10^9/L$.

VI. Quantitative disorders of basophils

 A. Basophilia
   1. Cause: Increased production by the bone marrow due to such disorders as hypersensitivity or myeloproliferative diseases.
   2. Laboratory evaluation: The direct basophil count is greater than $0.3 \times 10^9/L$.
 B. Basopenia
   1. Cause: Decreased production may occur during stress and infections.
   2. Laboratory evaluation: Decreased basophil counts are difficult to determine since the normal range is extremely low.

VII. Qualitative disorders of granulocytes
 A. Degenerative changes
   1. Döhle bodies
      a. Cause: Bacterial infections may cause neutrophils to mature faster than normal. Possibly, the hurried development causes residual RNA in the cytoplasm of the mature neutrophil.
      b. Laboratory evaluation: The peripheral blood smear reveals pale-blue–staining areas within the neutrophil cytoplasm.
   2. Pyknotic nucleus
      a. Cause: Bacterial infections may result in neutrophils that are near death.
      b. Laboratory evaluation: The peripheral blood smear reveals neutrophils with condensed round nuclei or nuclear fragments. Since pyknosis also may be due to prolonged contact between neutrophils and ethylenediaminetetraacetic acid (EDTA), fresh smears must be evaluated.
   3. Toxic granulation
      a. Cause: Bacterial infections induce the neutrophils to increase production of primary granules containing lysozymes.
      b. Laboratory evaluation: The peripheral blood smear reveals small, dark-staining granules within the cytoplasm of neutrophils.
   4. Toxic vacuoles
      a. Cause: As bacteria are phagocytized and digested by neutrophils, vacuoles appear in the cytoplasm.
      b. Laboratory evaluation: The peripheral blood smear reveals "holes" in the cytoplasm of neutrophils. Since vacuoles also may be due to prolonged contact between neutrophils and EDTA, fresh smears must be evaluated.

5. Lupus erythematosus (LE) cell
   a. Cause: When WBC nuclei are extruded from cells, they may be lysed by antinuclear antibody present in the individual with lupus. The resulting nuclear material is then engulfed by neutrophils.
   b. Laboratory evaluation: A LE preparation reveals neutrophils that have engulfed homogeneous nuclear masses. As a result, the nucleus of the neutrophil is pushed to the periphery of the cell and the phagocytized nucleus occupies most of the cytoplasmic area. Alternatively, the homogeneous mass may be surrounded by numerous neutrophils forming a rosette.

B. Nuclear changes
   1. Neutrophil hypersegmentation
      a. Cause: Interference with DNA synthesis from chemotherapy, B_{12} deficiency, or folate deficiency may cause segmented neutrophils to be hypersegmented. Hypersegmentation also may be a benign inherited disorder.
      b. Laboratory evaluation: The peripheral blood smear reveals segmented neutrophils with more than five lobes.
   2. Pelger-Huët anomaly (neutrophil hyposegmentation)
      a. Cause
         (1) Autosomal dominant inheritance of an abnormal gene produces mature granulocytes with bi-lobed and non-segmented condensed nuclei. The disorder results in a benign syndrome.
         (2) Bi-lobed and non-segmented neutrophils may be acquired in myeloproliferative disorders.
      b. Laboratory evaluation
         (1) Peripheral blood smear: Bi-lobed and non-segmented neutrophils, eosinophils, and basophils resemble a "shift to the left." A "pince-nez" appearance may be evident.
         (2) WBC count
            (a) Inherited: Normal
            (b) Acquired: Variable
   3. Nuclear appendages
      a. Cause: Drumstick appendages on neutrophils are thought to be an in-

activated X chromosome. Abnormal numbers may be seen in Klinefelter syndrome.
   b. Laboratory evaluation
      (1) Peripheral blood smear: The nuclei of numerous segmented neutrophils possess drumstick-shaped appendages.
      (2) Karyotyping: An extra X chromosome is seen in Klinefelter syndrome.

C. Cytoplasmic changes
   1. Alder-Reilly anomaly
      a. Cause: Autosomal recessive inheritance of an abnormal gene prevents the normal breakdown of mucopolysaccharides. The result is deposition of the mucopolysaccharides in the cytoplasm of neutrophils and monocytes.
      b. Laboratory evaluation: The peripheral blood smear reveals non-transient dark-staining granules in the granulocytes. These granules may be confused with toxic granulation.
   2. Auer bodies
      a. Cause: Primary granules may aggregate in myeloblasts and monoblasts during acute leukemias.
      b. Laboratory evaluation.
         (1) Peripheral blood smear: Myeloblasts or monoblasts may show red-staining rods in the cytoplasm.
         (2) Peroxidase stain: Auer bodies will stain positively.
   3. Chédiak-Higashi syndrome
      a. Cause: Autosomal recessive inheritance of an abnormal gene produces large lysosomes that cannot release their contents for bacterial digestion.
      b. Laboratory evaluation.
         (1) Peripheral blood smear: Large acidophilic granules are present in the cytoplasm of WBCs.
         (2) WBC count: Decreased.
   4. May-Hegglin anomaly
      a. Cause: Autosomal dominant inheritance of an abnormal gene causes pale-blue inclusions in the neutrophils. Giant platelets are also present.
      b. Laboratory evaluation: The peripheral blood smear reveals Döhle-like bodies in the neutrophils. Large, bizarre-shaped platelets are seen.

D. Artifactual changes
  1. Due to anticoagulant
    a. Cytoplasmic vacuolization
      (1) Description: Neutrophils have "holes" in the cytoplasm.
      (2) Remedy: The smear should be re-made from a fresh specimen.
    b. Karyorrhexis
      (1) Description: The WBC nucleus is cloverleaf-shaped.
      (2) Remedy: The smear should be re-made from a fresh specimen.
    c. Platelet satellitism
      (1) Description: Platelets adhere to the periphery of neutrophils.
      (2) Remedy: The smear should be re-made from a specimen collected in an anticoagulant other than EDTA.
    d. Pyknotic nucleus
      (1) Description: The WBC nucleus is extremely condensed and rounded.
      (2) Remedy: The smear should be re-made from a fresh specimen.
  2. Due to Wright's stain
    a. Stain precipitate
      (1) Description: Dark granules are present on the smear and may be confused with toxic granulation or bacteria.
      (2) Remedy: The stain should be filtered or changed before using.
    b. Poor staining
      (1) Description: WBC nuclei may be pale-blue due to basic buffer or extremely dark-blue due to acidic buffer.
      (2) Remedy: The buffer pH should be adjusted to 7.0.
  3. Due to trauma while making the smear
    a. Smudge cells
      (1) Description: The cytoplasm of WBCs has been stripped away leaving basket-like nuclei. These cells are likely to be numerous in leukemic specimens.
      (2) Remedy: Albumin (22 percent) should be added to the blood before making the smear.
    b. Abnormal WBC distribution on the smear
      (1) Description: Large cells tend to be pulled to the edge of the wedge smear.
      (2) Remedy: Differentials should be performed in the central portion of the smear.

VIII. Qualitative disorders of eosinophils
  A. Degranulation
    1. Cause: Decreased granules may result during myeloproliferative syndromes.
    2. Laboratory evaluation: The peripheral blood smear reveals eosinophils with few granules.
  B. Vacuolization
    1. Cause: Unknown.
    2. Laboratory evaluation: The peripheral blood smear reveals "holes" in the cytoplasm of eosinophils.
  C. Hypersegmentation
    1. Cause: Multiple segments of the nucleus of the eosinophil may be seen in conditions noted under neutrophil hypersegmentation. (See Section VII B1.)
    2. Laboratory evaluation: The peripheral blood smear reveals more than three lobes in the nucleus of the eosinophil.

IX. Qualitative disorder of basophils—degranulation
  A. Cause: Antigen stimulation may result in fewer granules being present in the basophils.
  B. Laboratory evaluation: The peripheral blood smear reveals basophils with few dark-staining granules.

X. Laboratory tests useful in assessing leukopoiesis
  A. Total WBC count.
    1. Manual: Using the hemacytometer, diluting fluids, and a WBC pipet, the WBC count may be calculated.
    2. Automated: Electrical impedance and/or light scatter may be used to determine the WBC count.
  B. WBC differential/Wright's stain.
    1. Relative count: The percentage of each type of WBC is determined from a 100-cell count.
    2. Absolute count: The percentage of each type of WBC is multiplied by the total WBC count.
    3. Assessment of abnormal morphology: Abnormalities of the WBC nucleus and/or cytoplasm should be noted.
  C. Correction for nucleated RBCs:

$$\frac{\text{Total WBC count} \times 100}{100 + \text{number of NRBCs per 100 WBCs}}$$

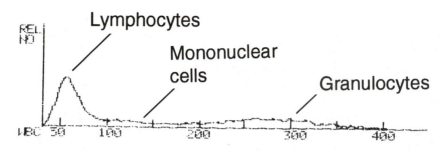

Femtoliters

D. WBC histogram: Broad categories of WBC types may be distinguished.
E. Direct eosinophil count: Eosinophils may be stained and counted on a hemacytometer.
F. Direct basophil count: Basophils may be stained and counted on a hemacytometer.
G. LE preparation: The presence of antinuclear antibody may be detected by the presence of phagocytized homogeneous nuclear material.
H. Thorn test: When ACTH is administered, the eosinophil count should decrease. Failure to decrease may indicate adrenocortical disease.

REFERENCES

Harmening: 30–34, 72–73, 241–253, 523–529, 545–551, 554–567
Lotspeich-Steininger: 288–299, 317–343, 356–359
McKenzie: 51–61, 251–268
Turgeon: 129–139, 144–150, 312, 343–347

Chapter 9

❦

Leukopoiesis: The Monocytes

I. Developmental changes
   A. Monoblast: The diameter is 12 to 20 micrometers. Occupying most of the cell, the nucleus has a fine chromatin pattern with several nucleoli.
   B. Promonocyte: The diameter is 14 to 18 micrometers. The large nucleus has a foamy appearance. Nucleoli may or may not be seen. The cytoplasm is blue-gray.
   C. Monocyte: The diameter is 12 to 20 micrometers. The nucleus appears foamy and folded. It may be rounded, elongated, or horseshoe-shaped. The abundant cytoplasm is gray with dust-like granules and a few vacuoles.
   D. Tissue macrophage: The diameter is 20 to 50 micrometers. A round or kidney-shaped nucleus with nucleoli is surrounded by voluminous cytoplasm. The cytoplasm may contain granules and vacuoles.

II. Kinetics: The cell matures within the bone marrow, crosses into the sinusoidal spaces, and eventually moves into the peripheral blood. Like the neutrophil, the monocyte enters the tissues by diapedesis. In the tissue, the monocyte transforms into a tissue macrophage and may live for months to years.

III. Functions
   A. Monocytes ingest particles of molecular to cellular size in an effort to protect the body. Antigenic material is processed so that the information can be transferred to lymphocytes for future reactions.
   B. Monocytes undergo continuous surveillance for tumor cells.
   C. Monocytes phagocytize dying cells and cellular by-products.

IV. Quantitative disorders of monocytes
   A. Monocytosis

   1. Cause: Increased production and release from the bone marrow due to such disorders as tuberculosis, chronic bacterial or parasitic infections, myeloproliferative states, post-chemotherapy, and hemolytic anemias.
   2. Laboratory evaluation: The absolute monocyte count is greater than 0.9×10^9/L.
   B. Monocytopenia
   1. Cause: Overpowering infections and administration of glucocorticoids may produce a decrease in monocytes.
   2. Laboratory evaluation: The absolute monocyte count is less than 0.2×10^9/L.

V. Qualitative disorders of monocytes
   A. Erythrophagocytosis
   1. Cause: Autoimmune hemolytic anemia causes increased phagocytosis of cells.
   2. Laboratory evaluation: The peripheral blood smear reveals monocytes with engulfed RBCs within the cytoplasm.
   B. Gaucher's disease
   1. Cause: Autosomal recessive inheritance of an enzyme deficiency results in the monocyte's inability to degrade glucocerebrosides.
   2. Laboratory evaluation.
      a. Peripheral blood smear: Normocytic, normochromic RBC morphology with pancytopenia.
      b. Bone marrow aspiration and biopsy: Gaucher's cells (large macrophages with wrinkled-looking cytoplasm and small, off-centered nucleus) are present.
      c. Acid phosphatase: Increased.
   C. Niemann-Pick disease
   1. Cause: Autosomal recessive inheritance of an enzyme deficiency results in the mon-

ocyte's inability to degrade sphingomyelin and cholesterol.
2. Laboratory evaluation.
   a. Peripheral blood smear: Monocytes and lymphocytes may show vacuoles.
   b. Bone marrow aspiration and biopsy: Niemann-Pick cells (large macrophages with foamy-looking cytoplasm) are present.
D. Sea-blue histiocytosis
1. Cause: The exact cause of sea-blue histiocytes is unknown, but it is thought to be an autosomal recessive inheritance of an enzyme deficiency resulting in lipid accumulation within the macrophage.
2. Laboratory evaluation.
   a. Platelet count: Decreased.
   b. Bone marrow aspiration and biopsy: Sea-blue histiocytes (large macrophages with blue-green cytoplasm) are present.
E. Tay-Sachs disease
1. Cause: Autosomal recessive inheritance of an enzyme deficiency results in cells engorged with undegraded ganglioside.

2. Laboratory evaluation.
   a. Peripheral blood smear: Lymphocytes contain vacuoles.
   b. Bone marrow aspiration and biopsy: Histiocytes with vacuoles are present.
F. Mucopolysaccharidoses
1. Cause: A group of related disorders develops as a result of various enzyme deficiencies. The respective deficiencies cause a failure of mucopolysaccharide degradation.
2. Laboratory evaluation.
   a. Peripheral blood smear: Leukocytes have Alder-Reilly granules.
   b. Tissue biopsy: Cells enlarged by unmetabolized mucopolysaccharides are seen.

REFERENCES

Harmening: 34–35, 403–411
Lotspeich-Steininger: 291, 299–301, 343–344, 359–361
McKenzie: 61–65, 233–236
Turgeon: 132–139, 144–145, 147, 150

Chapter 10

❧

Leukopoiesis: The Lymphocytes and the Plasma Cells

I. Developmental changes
  A. Lymphoid stem cell: The diameter is 12 to 20 micrometers. The large, round nucleus is finely reticulated and evenly stained. Nucleoli are visible. The scant cytoplasm is deep-blue.
  B. Prolymphocyte: The diameter is 15 to 18 micrometers. The nucleus occupies most of the cell. Some chromatin clumping renders nucleoli less visible.
  C. Normal lymphocyte.
    1. Small: The diameter is 6 to 10 micrometers. The cell is round to oval with a round to kidney-shaped nucleus that occupies the majority of the cell. Nucleoli may be present, but dense chromatin clumping precludes distinction. The scant cytoplasm is medium-blue.
    2. Large: The diameter is 11 to 18 micrometers. The cell frequently has an irregular outline. The nucleus may be round, oval, or indented with clumped chromatin. The moderate amount of cytoplasm is pale- to medium-blue and may scallop around adjacent RBCs. Some azurophilic granules may be present in the cytoplasm. These cells may be confused with monocytes that usually do not scallop around RBCs.
  D. Variant lymphocyte: The diameter is 15 to 27 micrometers. The nucleus may be round to convoluted, and the chromatin pattern may be fine to coarsely clumped. Nucleoli may be seen. Abundant blue cytoplasm often scallops around adjacent RBCs. These cells may also be confused with monocytes. Variant lymphocytes are also known as reactive lymphocytes, abnormal lymphocytes, immature lymphocytes, stimulated lymphocytes, atypical lymphocytes, Downey cells, and virocytes.
  E. Plasmacytoid lymphocyte: The diameter is 9 to 20 micrometers. Cell shape is round to oval with the nucleus slightly off center. A moderate amount of deep-blue cytoplasm encircles the nucleus and frequently exhibits a small perinuclear clear zone.
  F. Plasma cell: The diameter is 12 to 24 micrometers. Most often the cell is oval with the long axis of the oval nucleus aligned perpendicular to the long axis of the cell. The nucleus is eccentrically placed in the cell. An adjacent perinuclear clear zone is present within the deep-blue cytoplasm.

II. Kinetics: Lymphoid stem cells migrate to the thymus (giving rise to T lymphocytes) or the bursal equivalent lymphoid tissue (giving rise to B lymphocytes). The T and B cells migrate to the lymph nodes where they proliferate and enter the lymphatic system. The cells enter the peripheral blood with the lymphatic fluid. Eventually, the lymphocytes migrate into the tissues and once again enter the lymphatic fluid for recirculation. Some lymphocytes cannot be identified as T or B cells, and thus are designated as non-T, non-B lymphocytes or natural killer cells. Typically, about 80 percent of lymphocytes in the peripheral circulation are T lymphocytes, and approximately 20 percent are B lymphocytes.

III. Functions
  A. T lymphocytes direct immune reactions through a variety of lymphokines.
    1. Helper T (CD4) lymphocytes assist mac-

rophages in the activation of B lymphocytes.

2. Suppressor T (CD8) lymphocytes limit cellular and humoral response in immunity.

3. Delayed hypersensitivity T lymphocytes produce lymphokines that attract macrophages to the site of infection and confine them to the infected area.

4. Cytotoxic T lymphocytes, contained in both helper and suppressor subsets, eliminate cells carrying specific antigens.

B. B lymphocytes transform, with the aid of T lymphocytes and macrophages, into plasma cells that produce antibodies.

1. Antibodies are identified by their corresponding heavy chain as follows:
   a. Alpha chains define IgA.
   b. Delta chains define IgD.
   c. Epsilon chains define IgE.
   d. Gamma chains define IgG.
   e. Mu chains define IgM.

2. Antibodies also contain one type of light chains, either kappa or lambda.

C. Natural killer cells lyse specific cells directly or by antibody–dependent cell-mediated cytolysis.

IV. Quantitative disorders of lymphocytes
   A. Lymphocytosis
      1. Reactive, other than mononucleosis
         a. Cause: Proliferation of lymphocytes may occur in early childhood, hypersensitivity reactions, and certain viral diseases.
         b. Laboratory evaluation.
            (1) Absolute lymphocyte count: Greater than 4.5×10^9/L
            (2) Peripheral blood smear: Often reveals greater than 10 percent variant lymphocytes

(3) Heterophile antibodies: Negative
(4) Epstein-Barr virus titer: Negative
(5) Cytomegalovirus titer: Negative

2. Reactive due to mononucleosis
   a. Cause: Proliferation of lymphocytes may occur during infection with Epstein-Barr virus or cytomegalovirus.
   b. Laboratory evaluation
      (1) Epstein-Barr virus/infectious mononucleosis
         (a) Absolute lymphocyte count: Greater than 4.5×10^9/L
         (b) Peripheral blood smear: Often reveals greater than 10 percent variant lymphocytes
         (c) Heterophile antibodies: Usually positive after 1 week
         (d) Epstein-Barr virus titer: Increased
         (e) Cytomegalovirus titer: Negative
      (2) Cytomegalovirus infection
         (a) Absolute lymphocyte count: Greater than 4.5×10^9/L
         (b) Peripheral blood smear: Often reveals greater than 10 percent variant lymphocytes
         (c) Heterophile antibodies: Negative
         (d) Epstein-Barr virus titer: Negative
         (e) Cytomegalovirus titer: Increased

3. Summary of laboratory differentiation of reactive lymphocytosis (see figure below)

B. Lymphocytopenia
   1. Cause: A decrease in the number of lymphocytes may occur in disorders such as immunologic deficiency disorders, aplastic anemia, and chemotherapy.
   2. Laboratory evaluation

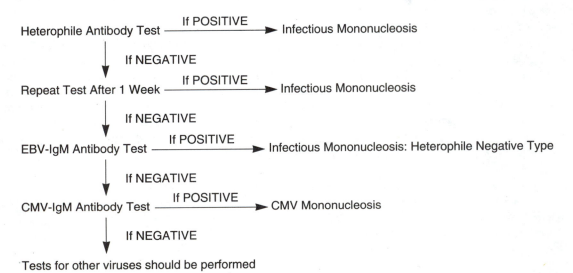

Heterophile Antibody Test ——— If POSITIVE ———→ Infectious Mononucleosis

If NEGATIVE

Repeat Test After 1 Week ——— If POSITIVE ———→ Infectious Mononucleosis

If NEGATIVE

EBV-IgM Antibody Test ——— If POSITIVE ———→ Infectious Mononucleosis: Heterophile Negative Type

If NEGATIVE

CMV-IgM Antibody Test ——— If POSITIVE ———→ CMV Mononucleosis

If NEGATIVE

Tests for other viruses should be performed

a. Absolute lymphocyte count: Less than 1.2×10^9/L
b. Absolute helper T lymphocyte count: Permanently decreased in AIDS

V. Qualitative disorders of lymphocytes
  A. Alder-Reilly granules
    1. Cause: Autosomal recessive inheritance of an abnormal gene prevents the normal breakdown of the mucopolysaccharides in the cytoplasm of lymphocytes, granulocytes, and monocytes.
    2. Laboratory evaluation: The peripheral blood smear reveals numerous coarse purple granules in the cytoplasm of lymphocytes, granulocytes, and monocytes.
  B. Chédiak-Higashi anomaly
    1. Cause: Autosomal recessive inheritance of an abnormal gene produces large lysosomes in lymphocytes and neutrophils.
    2. Laboratory evaluation: The peripheral blood smear reveals a single, large lavender granule in the cytoplasm of lymphocytes and multiple granules in neutrophilic cytoplasm.
  C. Reider clefts
    1. Cause: The cause and importance of this abnormality is undetermined at this time.
    2. Laboratory evaluation: The peripheral blood smear reveals a cleft in the lymphocyte nucleus.
  D. Smudge cells
    1. Cause: The cytoplasm of fragile or disintegrating lymphocytes may be pulled away from the cell during smear preparation. This is especially common in chronic lymphocytic leukemia.
    2. Laboratory evaluation: The peripheral blood smear reveals a bare reddish-purple–staining nucleus with no cytoplasm. Smudging may be prevented by adding 22 percent albumin to whole blood prior to smear preparation.
  E. Vacuoles
    1. Cause: Water-insoluble substances accumulate in the lymphocytic cytoplasm. The substances may be the result of an inherited disorder such as the mucopolysaccharidoses or acquired as in infectious mononucleosis.
    2. Laboratory evaluation: The peripheral blood smear reveals lymphocytes with ''holes'' in the cytoplasm created by dissolution of the contents by alcohol-based stains.

VI. Quantitative disorders of plasma cells—plasmacytosis
  1. Cause: An increase in plasma cell production may be the result of benign disorders, such as allergic states or viral and bacterial infections, or be the result of malignant disorders, such as multiple myeloma.
  2. Laboratory evaluation.
    a. Peripheral blood smear: RBC rouleaux is common, and occasional plasma cells may be seen.
    b. Bone marrow biopsy and aspirate: Numerous plasma cells may be seen.

VII. Qualitative disorders of plasma cells
  A. Flame cell
    1. Cause: The exact cause is unknown, but morphologic changes are due to increased amounts of glycoprotein within the plasma cell.
    2. Laboratory evaluation: Plasma cells in the bone marrow may display a pinkish-red cytoplasm instead of the typical deep-blue color.
  B. Polyploidy
    1. Cause: A few normal plasma cells as well as myeloma plasma cells may contain two or more nuclei.
    2. Laboratory evaluation: Plasma cells in the bone marrow display more than one nucleus.
  C. Russell bodies
    1. Cause: Under normal circumstances, a small amount of gamma globulins may accumulate within the cell. Large amounts may be seen in disorders such as multiple myeloma.
    2. Laboratory evaluation: Plasma cells in the bone marrow will show round to rod-shaped and colorless to purple inclusions.
  D. Mott cell
    1. Cause: Numerous Russell bodies may accumulate within the cell in disorders such as hypergammaglobulinemias and multiple myeloma.
    2. Laboratory evaluation: Plasma cells in the bone marrow may have a berry- or grape-like appearance as the cell looks stuffed with colorless to purple globules or rods.

REFERENCES

Harmening: 21–27, 35–37, 249–250, 408
Lotspeich-Steininger: 303–316, 348–355, 358–359, 477
McKenzie: 65–80, 267–275
Turgeon: 154–164, 168–181

Chapter 11

Myeloproliferative Disorders

I. General classification of leukemias is based on:
   A. Cell type
      1. Non-lymphocytic
         a. Myelocytic
         b. Monocytic
         c. Myelomonocytic
         d. Megakaryocytic
         e. Erythrocytic
      2. Lymphocytic
   B. Cell maturity
      1. Immature in acute leukemias
      2. Mature in chronic leukemias

II. Laboratory evaluation of neoplastic disorders
   A. Morphology
      1. Peripheral blood smear: Neoplastic cell is usually evident.
      2. Bone marrow biopsy and aspiration: The hypercellularity of the marrow frequently results in aspiration difficulties. Megaloblastic, erythropoietic, and sideroblastic disturbances may be evident.
   B. Cytogenetics: Chromosome deletions (loss of chromosomal segment) and translocations (segment detached from one chromosome is attached to another chromosome) are evaluated. The first chromosomal abnormality to be discovered was the Philadelphia (Ph') chromosome, which is associated with chronic myelocytic leukemia. Oncogenes exist in the inactive state. If activated, neoplastic transformation occurs.
   C. Special cytochemical stains
      1. Acid phosphatase: The enzyme is present in all blood cells, but most cells lose their positivity when treated with tartaric acid prior to staining. The notable exceptions are the cells of hairy cell leukemia and histiocytes.
      2. Esterase: The stain is useful in differen-

tiating between acute myelocytic leukemia and acute monocytic leukemia.
      a. Specific: The enzyme is present in granulocytic cells.
      b. Non-specific: The enzyme is present in the monocytic cell line, megakaryocytes, and some granulocytes. Alpha-naphthyl acetate or alpha-naphthyl butyrate may be used as a substrate with slightly different results.
   3. Leukocyte alkaline phosphatase (LAP): The enzyme is present in mature granulocytes and is useful in differentiating between chronic myelocytic leukemia and leukemoid reactions.
   4. Myeloperoxidase: The enzyme is present in myelocytic cells and, to a lesser extent, in monocytic cells. It is useful in differentiating between acute non-lymphocytic leukemia (ANLL) and acute lymphocytic leukemia (ALL) in fresh specimens.
   5. Periodic acid-Schiff: The glycogen in cells stains; therefore, most cells stain positively. The cells of a neoplastic lymphoid series and of erythroleukemia stain with block positivity.
   6. Sudan black B: Lipids in granulocytes, monocytes, megakaryocytes, and RBCs of erythroleukemia stain positively. It is useful in differentiating between ANLL and ALL in older specimens.
   7. Toluidine blue: Mucopolysaccharides of basophils and mast cells stain positively. It is useful for identification of basophilic leukemia and mast cell disease.
   D. Terminal deoxynucleotidyl transferase (TdT): The DNA polymerase is present in immature lymphocytes and is useful in distinguishing lymphoblastic disorders.
   E. Immunologic markers: The cell membrane

contains numerous distinctive antigens and receptors that identify cell types at various stages of development.

F. Muramidase: The enzyme normally is found in granulocytes and monocytes; however, the enzyme is markedly increased in acute monocytic leukemia.

G. Cerebrospinal fluid examination: Leukemic cells can multiply in the meninges since chemotherapeutic drugs do not cross the blood-brain barrier. Proliferation is especially common in ALL.

III. Myeloproliferative disorders
A. Acute disorders
1. Incidence.
a. Usually seen in adults
b. Slightly higher incidence in males
2. Cause: Evidence indicates that exposure to radiation or environmental mutagens, genetic predisposition, and possibly viral infection may induce malignant transformation of hematopoietic cells.
3. General physical findings: Well-nourished patient with pallor, petechiae, and complaints of fatigue.
4. Treatment: Cytotoxic chemotherapy, radiotherapy, and bone marrow transplantation.
5. French-American-British (FAB) classification.
a. M0
(1) Synonym: Acute undifferentiated leukemia
(2) Laboratory evaluation
(a) Peripheral blood smear: Unclassified blast cells predominate.
(b) Cytochemical stains: Negative.
b. M1
(1) Synonym: Acute myelocytic leukemia without maturation
(2) Laboratory evaluation
(a) Peripheral blood smear: Almost all WBCs are blasts with very similar appearance. Auer rods may be seen.
(b) Bone marrow aspiration and biopsy. Hypercellular with at least 30 percent blasts.
(c) Myeloperoxidase: Positive.
(d) Sudan black B: Positive.
(e) Specific esterase: Positive.
(f) Cerebrospinal fluid examination: Negative.

c. M2
(1) Synonym: Acute myelocytic leukemia with maturation
(2) Laboratory evaluation
(a) Peripheral blood smear: At least 50 percent of the WBCs are blasts, but some mature granulocytes are also seen. Auer rods may be present as well.
(b) Bone marrow aspiration and biopsy: Hypercellular with at least 30 percent blasts plus at least 10 percent granulocytes.
(c) Myeloperoxidase: Positive.
(d) Sudan black B: Positive.
(e) Specific esterase: Positive.
(f) Cytogenetics: Translocation from chromosome 8q to 21q is sometimes seen.
d. M3
(1) Synonym: Acute promyelocytic leukemia
(2) Laboratory evaluation
(a) Peripheral blood smear: Numerous promyelocytes are present. Faggots of Auer rods and hypergranulation may be seen in the cytoplasm of malignant cells.
(b) Myeloperoxidase: Positive.
(c) Sudan black B: Positive.
(d) Specific esterase: Positive.
(e) Cytogenetics: Translocation from chromosome 17 to 15 is sometimes seen.
e. M4
(1) Synonym: Acute myelomonocytic leukemia
(2) Laboratory evaluation
(a) Peripheral blood smear: WBCs with convoluted nuclei predominate.
(b) Bone marrow aspiration and biopsy: At least 20 percent monocytes, 30 percent blasts, and 20 percent granulocytes are present.
(c) Myeloperoxidase: Positive.
(d) Sudan black B: Positive.
(e) Specific esterase: Positive.
(f) Non-specific esterase: Positive.
(g) Muramidase: Normal to elevated.

               (h) Cytogenetics: Chromosome 16 abnormalities.
       f. M5
          (1) Synonym: Acute monocytic leukemia
          (2) Laboratory evaluation
               (a) Peripheral blood smear: Immature monocytes predominate.
               (b) Bone marrow aspiration and biopsy: Monocytic cells predominate.
               (c) Myeloperoxidase: Negative to weakly positive.
               (d) Sudan black B: Negative to weakly positive.
               (e) Non-specific esterase: Positive.
               (f) Specific esterase: Negative.
               (g) Muramidase: Markedly increased.
               (h) Cytogenetics: Translocation from chromosome 9 to 11.
       g. M6
          (1) Synonym: Erythroleukemia
          (2) Laboratory evaluation
               (a) Peripheral blood smear: Normocytic, normochromic anemia with NRBCs, some blasts, and thrombocytopenia are seen.
               (b) Bone marrow aspiration and biopsy: Erythroid hyperplasia is created by the presence of at least 50 percent erythroid precursors. Greater than 30 percent non-erythroid blasts will be present.
       h. M7
          (1) Synonym: Acute megakaryocytic leukemia
          (2) Laboratory evaluation
               (a) Peripheral blood smear: Immature megakaryocytes and platelets are seen.
               (b) Platelet count: Normal to increased.
               (c) Non-specific esterase (alpha-naphthyl-butyrate): Negative.
               (d) Non-specific esterase (naphthol AS-D chloroacetate): Positive.
B. Myelodysplastic syndromes
  1. Incidence
    a. Usually seen in older adults.
    b. Higher occurrence is seen in males.

  2. Cause: The syndromes often develop following chemical, viral, and/or radiation exposure.
  3. General physical findings: Patients present with single or multiple findings of organomegaly, fatigue, recurrent infections, fever, and bleeding.
  4. Treatment: Supportive therapy until leukemia develops.
  5. FAB classification.
    a. Refractory anemia (RA) — Laboratory evaluation
       (1) Peripheral blood smear: Pelgeroid cells with rare blasts
       (2) WBC count: Normal to increased
       (3) Bone marrow aspiration and biopsy: Megaloblastoid changes with less than 5 percent blasts
       (4) Cytogenetics: Deletion of a part of the long arm of chromosome 5
    b. RA with ringed sideroblasts (RARS) — Laboratory evaluation
       (1) Peripheral blood smear: Di-morphic anemia with rare blasts
       (2) WBC count: Normal to decreased
       (3) Bone marrow aspiration and biopsy: At least 15 percent sideroblasts
       (4) Cytogenetics: Deletion of a part of the long arm of chromosome 5
    c. RA with excess blasts (RAEB) — Laboratory evaluation
       (1) Peripheral blood smear: Anemia with less than 5 percent blasts.
       (2) WBC count: Normal to decreased.
       (3) Bone marrow aspiration and biopsy: The marrow contains 5 to 20 percent blasts.
       (4) Cytogenetics: Deletion of a part of the long arm of chromosome 5.
    d. RAEB in transformation (RAEBIT) — Laboratory evaluation
       (1) Peripheral blood smear: At least 5 percent blasts are seen.
       (2) WBC count: Normal to decreased.
       (3) Bone marrow aspiration and biopsy: Twenty to thirty percent blasts.
       (4) Cytogenetics: Deletion of a part of the long arm of chromosome 5.
    e. Chronic myelomonocytic leukemia (CMMoL) — Laboratory evaluation
       (1) Peripheral blood smear: Persistent monocytosis with less than 5 percent blasts
       (2) WBC count: Increased

(3) Bone marrow aspiration and biopsy: Zero to twenty percent blasts

(4) Cytogenetics: Deletion of a part of the long arm of chromosome 12

C. Chronic disorders

1. Incidence: Usually seen after 40 years of age, except in juvenile chronic myelocytic leukemia

2. General physical findings: Hepatosplenomegaly and pallor

3. Classification

a. Polycythemia vera

(1) Laboratory evaluation

(a) WBC count: Moderately increased with left shift and basophilia.

(b) RBC count: Increased with rare NRBC.

(c) Platelet count: Increased.

(d) RBC mass: Increased.

(e) Erythropoietin level: Decreased to absent.

(f) Blood viscosity: Increased.

(g) LAP: Increased.

(h) Bone marrow aspiration and biopsy: Hypercellular with normal M : E ratio and increased number of megakaryocytes.

(i) Philadelphia chromosome: Absent.

(j) Coagulation studies: Since the patient's hematocrit is elevated, care must be taken to adjust the blood to anticoagulant ratio when collecting a specimen for testing. (See Chapter 14, Section VA.)

(2) Treatment: Therapeutic phlebotomy, radioactive phosphorus, and myelosuppressive drugs

b. Myeloid metaplasia

(1) Laboratory evaluation

(a) WBC count: Variable.

(b) RBC count: Decreased.

(c) Platelet count: Variable.

(d) LAP: Normal to increased.

(e) Bone marrow aspiration and biopsy: Hypocellular with fibrotic features.

(f) Peripheral blood smear: Leukoerythroblastosis. Morphology of RBCs shows dacryocytes (teardrop cells), ovalocytes, and polychromasia.

(g) Philadelphia chromosome: Absent.

(2) Treatment: Supportive

c. Essential thrombocythemia

(1) Laboratory evaluation

(a) WBC count: Slightly increased

(b) RBC count: Normal to slightly increased

(c) Platelet count: Markedly increased

(d) LAP: Normal to increased

(e) Bone marrow aspiration and biopsy: Megakaryocytic hyperplasia

(f) Peripheral blood smear: Numerous platelets with bizarre size and shape

(g) Philadelphia chromosome: Absent

(2) Treatment: Supportive

d. Chronic myelocytic leukemia

(1) Laboratory evaluation

(a) WBC count: Moderately to markedly increased.

(b) RBC count: Normal to decreased.

(c) Platelet count: Variable.

(d) LAP: Low to absent.

(e) Bone marrow aspiration and biopsy: Hypercellular with predominance of granulocytes.

(f) Peripheral blood smear: Metamyelocytes and mature granulocytes predominate but blasts may be seen.

(g) Philadelphia chromosome: Present in the majority of cases. Presence of the Philadelphia chromosome indicates a better prognosis and response to therapy.

(2) Treatment: Chemotherapy and bone marrow transplantation

e. Juvenile chronic myelocytic leukemia

(1) Laboratory evaluation

(a) WBC count: Slightly to moderately increased

(b) RBC count: Decreased

(c) Platelet count: Decreased

(d) LAP: Decreased

(e) Peripheral blood smear: Numerous granulocytic precursors, but less than 10 percent blasts

(f) Muramidase: Increased
(g) Philadelphia chromosome: Absent
(2) Treatment: Chemotherapy and bone marrow transplantation

IV. Side effects of treatment for leukemia
A. Anemia: The therapeutic drugs are toxic to normal as well as abnormal cells. In addition, malignant cells crowd normal cells out of the marrow.
B. Hemorrhage: Platelets also are decreased leading to an increased bleeding tendency.

C. Infections: The immune system is compromised by the chemotherapy.
D. Urate nephropathy: As the masses of abnormal cells are degraded, uric acid levels increase. The uric acid may precipitate in the kidney causing renal dysfunction.

REFERENCES

Harmening: 266–282, 292–311, 326–365
Lotspeich-Steininger: 379–393, 408–446
McKenzie: 277–337
Turgeon: 186–191, 194–209, 224–241, 248–259

Chapter 12

Lymphoproliferative Disorders

I. The normal lymph node
  A. Structure
    1. Cortex: B lymphocytes populate the outermost region.
    2. Paracortex: T lymphocytes populate the region between the cortex and the medulla.
    3. Medulla: B lymphocytes and plasma cells populate the innermost region.

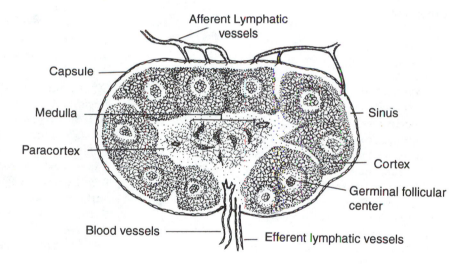

  B. Function
    1. Production of lymphocytes
    2. Filtration of lymphatic fluid

II. Lymphoblastic disorders
  A. Acute disorders
    1. Incidence: Usually seen in childhood.
    2. General physical findings: The patient presents with fatigue, lymphadenopathy, pallor, and sometimes fever and petechiae.
    3. Treatment: Chemotherapy, radiotherapy, and bone marrow transplantation.
    4. FAB classification.
      a. L1
        (1) Synonym: Acute lymphocytic leukemia (ALL) of childhood

        (2) Laboratory evaluation
          (a) WBC count: Usually increased.
          (b) RBC count: Markedly decreased.
          (c) Platelet count: Markedly decreased.
          (d) Peripheral blood smear: Homogeneous small blasts predominate.
          (e) Bone marrow aspiration and biopsy: Hypercellular.
          (f) Myeloperoxidase: Negative.
          (g) Sudan black B: Negative.
          (h) Periodic acid-Schiff: Large block positivity.
          (i) Terminal deoxynucleotidyl transferase (TdT): Positive.

b. L2
  (1) Synonym: ALL of adulthood
  (2) Laboratory evaluation
      (a) WBC count: Usually increased.
      (b) RBC count: Markedly decreased.
      (c) Platelet count: Markedly decreased.
      (d) Peripheral blood smear: Heterogeneous large blasts predominate.
      (e) Bone marrow aspiration and biopsy: Hypercellular.
      (f) Myeloperoxidase: Negative.
      (g) Sudan black B: Negative.
      (h) Periodic acid-Schiff: Weak block positivity.
      (i) TdT: Positive.
c. L3
  (1) Synonym: Leukemia of Burkitt's type.
  (2) Laboratory evaluation.
      (a) WBC count: Usually increased.
      (b) RBC count: Markedly decreased.
      (c) Platelet count: Markedly decreased.
      (d) Peripheral blood smear: Homogeneous blasts with vacuoles and deep-blue cytoplasm predominate.
      (e) Bone marrow aspiration and biopsy: Hypercellular.
      (f) Myeloperoxidase: Negative.
      (g) Sudan black B: Negative.
      (h) Specific and non-specific esterases: Negative.
      (i) Periodic acid-Schiff: Positive.
      (j) TdT: Positive.
      (k) Cytogenetics: Frequent translocation from chromosome 2, 14, or 22 to chromosome 8.
5. Immunologic classification.
  a. Common ALL — laboratory evaluation
    (1) Common ALL antigen (CALLA): Positive
    (2) T-cell markers: Negative
    (3) B-cell markers: Positive
    (4) Surface immunoglobulin: Negative
    (5) Cytoplasmic immunoglobulin: Negative
    (6) TdT: Positive
  b. Pre-T ALL — laboratory evaluation
    (1) E rosettes: Negative
    (2) T-cell markers: Positive
    (3) TdT: Positive
  c. Pre-B ALL — laboratory evaluation
    (1) CALLA: Positive
    (2) T-cell markers: Negative
    (3) B-cell markers: Positive
    (4) Surface immunoglobulin: Negative
    (5) Cytoplasmic immunoglobulin: Positive
    (6) TdT: Positive
  d. Null ALL — laboratory evaluation
    (1) CALLA: Negative
    (2) T-cell markers: Negative
    (3) B-cell markers: Negative
    (4) Surface immunoglobulin: Negative
    (5) Cytoplasmic immunoglobulin: Negative
    (6) TdT: Negative
  e. T ALL — laboratory evaluation
    (1) CALLA: Negative
    (2) E rosettes: Positive
    (3) T-cell markers: Positive
    (4) B-cell markers: Negative
    (5) Surface immunoglobulin: Negative
    (6) Cytoplasmic immunoglobulin: Negative
    (7) TdT: Positive
  f. B ALL — laboratory evaluation
    (1) CALLA: Usually negative
    (2) T-cell markers: Negative
    (3) B-cell markers: Positive
    (4) Surface immunoglobulin: Positive
    (5) Cytoplasmic immunoglobulin: Positive
    (6) TdT: Negative
B. Chronic disorders
  1. Incidence
    a. The disease usually occurs in middle-aged to older adults.
    b. A higher occurrence is seen in males.
  2. General physical findings: The patient may be asymptomatic or exhibit fatigue on exertion.
  3. Treatment: Chemotherapy and radiotherapy.
  4. Classification.
    a. Chronic lymphocytic leukemia (CLL) — laboratory evaluation
      (1) WBC count: Moderately to severely elevated with persistent lymphocytosis in excess of 5×10^9/L.
      (2) RBC count: Usually normal until terminal stages of the disorder.

(3) Platelet count: Usually normal until terminal stages of the disorder.

(4) Peripheral blood smear: Small lymphocytes produce a monotonous picture. Smudge cells may be numerous unless albumin is added to the blood prior to preparing the blood smear.

(5) Bone marrow aspiration and biopsy: Hypercellular with at least 30 percent "mature" lymphocytes.

(6) B lymphocyte markers: Usually positive.

(7) Direct antiglobulin test: Frequently positive.

(8) Cytogenetics: Trisomy 12 is often present.

b. Prolymphocytic leukemia (PLL) — laboratory evaluation

(1) WBC count: Increased

(2) RBC count: Normal to decreased

(3) Platelet count: Normal to decreased

(4) Peripheral blood smear: Small to large number of prolymphocytes

(5) Bone marrow aspiration and biopsy: Hypercellularity due to prolymphocyte predominance

c. Hairy cell leukemia — laboratory evaluation

(1) WBC count: Normal to decreased.

(2) RBC count: Decreased.

(3) Platelet count: Decreased.

(4) Peripheral blood smear: Mononuclear cells with cytoplasmic hair-like projections are evident.

(5) Bone marrow aspiration and biopsy: Fibrosis is often present.

(6) B lymphocyte markers: Positive.

(7) Tartrate-resistant acid phosphatase: Positive.

C. Lymphomas

1. General physical findings: A swollen painless lymph node is felt.

2. Treatment: Chemotherapy and radiotherapy.

3. Classification is based on lymph node structure, cell predominance, and cell differentiation.

a. Hodgkin's disease

(1) Incidence

(a) A high rate of occurrence develops in late adolescence and in late adulthood.

(b) A higher occurrence is seen in males.

(2) Laboratory evaluation

(a) WBC count: Normal to increased.

(b) RBC count: Normal to decreased.

(c) Platelet count: Normal.

(d) Peripheral blood smear: Monocytosis and eosinophilia may be seen.

(e) Lymph node biopsy/Rye classification.

(i) Diffuse lymphocyte predominance: Numerous lymphocytes in a diffuse pattern and rare Reed-Sternberg cells

(ii) Nodular sclerosis: Moderate number of lymphocytes and few Reed-Sternberg cells in nodules

(iii) Mixed cellularity: Diffuse infiltrate of lymphocytes, granulocytes, and plasma cells, in addition to a moderate number of Reed-Sternberg cells

(iv) Lymphocyte depletion: Diffuse pattern of fibrosis with numerous Reed-Sternberg cells

b. Non-Hodgkin's lymphoma

(1) Incidence

(a) The disease is more predominant in middle-aged to older adults.

(b) Occurrence is more frequent in males than females.

(2) Laboratory evaluation

(a) WBC count: Normal

(b) RBC count: Normal

(c) Platelet count: Normal

(d) Lymph node biopsy/international working formulation

(i) Low grade: Small to large lymphocytes slowly infiltrating the lymph node

(ii) Intermediate grade: Small to large lymphocytes progressively infiltrating the lymph node

(iii) High grade: Small to large lymphocytes rap-

idly infiltrating the lymph node
c. Sézary syndrome—non-Hodgkin's lymphoma
  (1) Incidence
    (a) Older adults have a higher incidence of the syndrome.
    (b) More males than females have the syndrome.
    (c) The syndrome usually follows a history of mycosis fungoides.
  (2) Laboratory evaluation
    (a) Peripheral blood smear: Large, bizarre cells with cerebriform nuclei are present.
    (b) CD4 markers: Positive.

III. Plasma cell disorders
  A. Multiple myeloma
    1. General physical findings: An afebrile, middle-aged to older patient presents with skeletal pain and pallor.
    2. Treatment: Chemotherapy and radiotherapy.
    3. Laboratory evaluation.
      a. WBC count: Normal to low.
      b. RBC count: Decreased.
      c. Platelet count: Usually normal.
      d. Peripheral blood smear: Rouleaux.
      e. Bone marrow aspiration and biopsy: At least 10 to 30 percent plasma cells. Mott cells, flame cells, and plasma cells with Russell bodies and immunoglobulin crystals may be seen.
      f. Serum protein electrophoresis: Monoclonal peak.
      g. Immunoelectrophoresis: Elevation of IgA, IgD, IgE, IgG, or IgM.
      h. Bence-Jones protein: Often positive.
      i. Blood viscosity: Increased.
  B. Waldenström's macroglobulinemia
    1. General physical findings: The patient is usually an older male with complaints of weakness, fatigue, and abnormal bleeding.
    2. Treatment: Plasmapheresis and chemotherapy.
    3. Laboratory evaluation.
      a. WBC count: Normal.
      b. RBC count: Decreased.
      c. Platelet count: Normal.
      d. Peripheral blood smear: Rouleaux.
      e. Bone marrow aspiration and biopsy: Small lymphocytes with plasmacytoid features are seen. Mast cells may also be increased.
      f. Serum protein electrophoresis: Monoclonal peak.
      g. Immunoelectrophoresis: Elevated IgM.
      h. Coagulation studies: Frequently abnormal.
      i. Blood viscosity: Increased.
      j. Cryoglobulins: Positive.
  C. Plasma cell leukemia
    1. General physical findings: The patient presents with organomegaly and abnormal bleeding.
    2. Treatment: Chemotherapy.
    3. Laboratory evaluation.
      a. WBC count: Decreased.
      b. RBC count: Decreased.
      c. Platelet count: Decreased.
      d. Peripheral blood smear: Plasma cells and a leukoerythroblastic picture are revealed.
      e. Bone marrow aspiration and biopsy: Numerous plasma cells.
  D. Heavy chain diseases
    1. General physical findings: The patient presents with fever, pallor, and recurrent infections.
    2. Treatment: Chemotherapy.
    3. Laboratory evaluation.
      a. WBC count: Increased
      b. RBC count: Decreased
      c. Platelet count: Normal to decreased
      d. Peripheral blood smear: Eosinophilia and sometimes plasmacytosis
      e. Serum protein electrophoresis: Hypogammaglobulinemia with a broad band in the beta-gamma region

IV. Immune deficiency disorders
  A. Congenital agammaglobulinemia—laboratory evaluation
    1. B lymphocyte count: Decreased
    2. Lymph node biopsy: Decreased number of plasma cells
    3. Immunoglobulin assays: Decreased
  B. AIDS
    1. General physical findings: The patient presents with weakness, unexplained weight loss, fever, swollen lymph nodes, and opportunistic infections.
    2. Laboratory evaluation.
      a. HIV antibody: Positive
      b. Helper T lymphocyte (CD4) count: Decreased
      c. WBC count: Decreased
      d. RBC count: Decreased
      e. Platelet count: Decreased

REFERENCES

Harmening: 230–231, 282–291, 312–326, 366–402
Lotspeich-Steininger: 448–480, 684–685
McKenzie: 273–275, 337–362
Turgeon: 198–205, 209, 213–220, 223–241

Section Two Worksheets

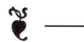

1. Blood is pipetted to the 0.5 mark of the WBC pipet, and the number of cells counted in the standard WBC squares equals 475 WBCs. Calculate the WBC count.

2. A. Blood is pipetted to the 1.0 mark of the WBC pipet, and the number of eosinophils counted in nine primary squares equals 53. Calculate the eosinophil count.

   B. The patient in part A had a WBC count of 10.0×10^9/L, and the differential revealed 6% eosinophils. Calculate the absolute eosinophil count.

C. Determine whether the accuracy of the first count (part A) is verified by the second calculation (part B). Should the count be reported or repeated?

3. A differential leukocyte count revealed 20 nucleated RBCs per 100 WBCs. The total leukocyte count was 21.0×10^9/L. Calculate the corrected total leukocyte count.

4. A complete blood count on a patient reveals the following data:

WBC ($\times 10^9$/L): 15.0
Differential:

Segmented neutrophils	80%
Band neutrophils	5%
Lymphocytes	13%
Monocytes	1%
Eosinophils	1%

Calculate the absolute cell count for each type of cell and give the appropriate relative and absolute terminology such as relative neutropenia, absolute neutrophilia, etc.

A. Absolute neutrophil count

B. Neutrophil terminology

C. Absolute lymphocyte count

D. Lymphocyte terminology

E. Absolute monocyte count

F. Monocyte terminology

G. Absolute eosinophil count

H. Eosinophil terminology

5. Label the Coulter WBC histogram by identifying the cells found in each location.

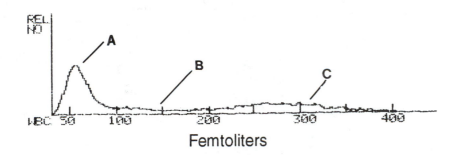

6. Label the Coulter VCS WBC scattergram by identifying the cells found in each location.

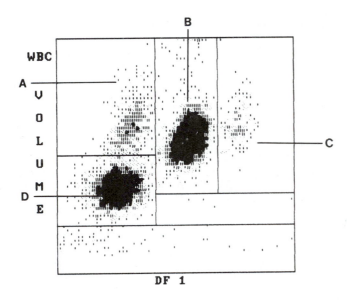

7. Label the Technicon H·1 WBC/peroxidase cytogram by identifying the cells found in each location.

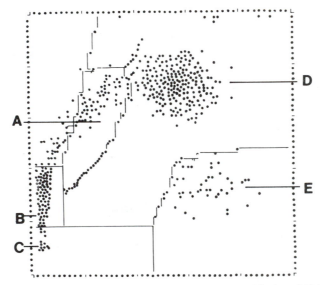

Adapted from Brown BA. *Hematology: Principles and Procedures*, ed 5. Philadelphia. Lea & Febiger, 1988, p. 388 with permission.

8. Label the Technicon H·1 basophil lobularity cytogram by identifying the cells found in each location.

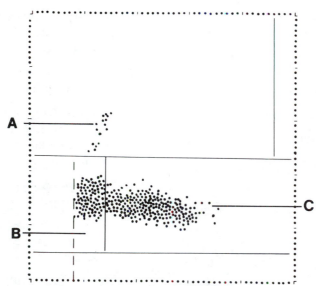

Adapted from Brown BA. *Hematology: Principles and Procedures*, ed 5. Philadelphia. Lea & Febiger, 1988, p. 389 with permission.

9. Define the following:

   A. Colony-stimulating factor

   B. Marginating cells

   C. Left shift

   D. Toxic granulation

   E. Döhle bodies

   F. Phagocytosis

   G. Neutropenia

10. Match the neutrophilic abnormality on the left with the appropriate description on the right. Each description may be used only once.

A. _____ Cyclic neutropenia

B. _____ Chédiak-Higashi disease

C. _____ May-Hegglin anomaly

D. _____ Pelger-Huët anomaly

E. _____ Chronic granulomatous disease

F. _____ Bacterial infection

G. _____ Alder-Reilly anomaly

a. Neutrophilia with a left shift, toxic granulation, Döhle bodies, and cytoplasmic vacuolization

b. Decreased circulating granulocytes recurring about every 21–28 days

c. Autosomal recessive disorder manifesting itself with large lysosomal inclusions in all types of leukocytes, recurrent infections, and hypopigmentation

d. Neutrophilic hyposegmentation; "pince-nez" cells

e. Mucopolysaccharidoses associated with dark-staining, coarse cytoplasmic granules in leukocytes

f. Neutrophils with blue-staining inclusions that resemble Döhle bodies

g. Segmented neutrophils with more than five lobes

h. Phagocytic cells are unable to digest microorganisms following ingestion

11. State the stages of neutrophil development from the least mature to the most mature.

12. Identify the WBC from the following description on a Wright's-stained smear.

A. A round cell with a nucleus that is slightly indented (kidney-shaped). The chromatin is moderately clumped and no nucleoli are visible. Numerous secondary pinkish granules fill the buff-colored cytoplasm.

B. A small, round cell with scant blue cytoplasm. The nucleus is round and coarsely clumped with no or indistinct nucleoli visible.

C. A motile cell with a bi-lobed nucleus. The chromatin is coarsely clumped. Many reddish-orange granules populate the cytoplasm.

D. A cell with a moderate amount of bluish nongranular cytoplasm. The nucleus is round with a finely reticulated chromatin pattern and distinct nucleoli.

E. A large cell with voluminous blue cytoplasm that indents when in contact with RBCs. The nucleus is slightly oval and moderately clumped with a nucleolus present.

F. A large cell with abundant grayish cytoplasm that does not indent when in contact with RBCs. The light-lavender nucleus is folded with a lacy or ground-glass appearance.

G. An oval cell with deep-blue cytoplasm and a perinuclear clear zone. The nucleus is eccentric and oval with the long axis perpendicular to the long axis of the cell.

13. Match the disease on the left with the appropriate enzyme deficiency on the right. Each response may be used only once.

A. _____ Gaucher's disease   a. Hexosaminidase

B. _____ Niemann-Pick disease   b. Beta-glucocerebrosidase

C. _____ Tay-Sachs disease   c. Sphingomyelinase

14. State the functions of each of the following cells.

A. Neutrophils

B. Eosinophils

C. Basophils

    D. Monocytes

    E. Lymphocytes

    F. Plasma cells

15. Interpret the following laboratory data on patients suspected of having infectious mononucleosis. Choices are:

    a. Infectious mononucleosis without liver involvement
    b. Infectious mononucleosis with liver involvement
    c. CMV mononucleosis without liver involvement
    d. CMV mononucleosis with liver involvement
    e. Reactive lymphocytosis due to other causes
    f. No hematologic abnormality

Laboratory Test	Patient A	Patient B	Patient C
Patient data	18-year-old male	22-year-old female	64-year-old male
CBC	WBC: elevated with 65% abnormal and immature lymphocytes	WBC: normal with 90% reactive lymphocytes	WBC: elevated with 73% reactive lymphocytes
Heterophile antibody test	Negative	Positive	Negative
EBV antibody test	Negative	1:512	Negative
CMV antibody test	Negative	Negative	1:256
Liver enzymes	Normal	Normal	Elevated
Interpretation			

16. Name the five classes of immunoglobulins.

17. Match the FAB classification on the left with the appropriate acute myeloid leukemia on the right. Each answer may be used only once.

    A. _____ M1   a. Erythroleukemia

    B. _____ M2   b. Megakaryocytic

    C. _____ M3   c. Monocytic

    D. _____ M4   d. Myelomonocytic

    E. _____ M5   e. Promyelocytic

    F. _____ M6   f. Myeloblastic with maturation

    G. _____ M7   g. Myeloblastic without maturation

18. Complete the following chart by naming the constituent of the cell that is stained by the cytochemical stain, the type of cell that usually stains positive, and when the stain would be used (or the expected results). The first stain is completed as an example.

Leukocyte Special Stains			
Special Stains	Constituent Stained	Cell Type Stained	Results/ Comments
Leukocyte alkaline phosphatase (LAP)	Enzyme: LAP	Neutrophils	Increased in pregnancy, polycythemia vera, infections, leukemoid reaction, and CML blast crisis. Decreased in CML, PNH, sideroblastic anemia, secondary polycythemia, and sickle cell anemia.
Myeloperoxidase			
Specific esterase (naphthol AS-D chloroacetate)			
Non-specific esterase (alpha-naphthyl butyrate)			
Combined esterase			
Tartrate-resistant acid phosphatase (TRAP)			
Sudan black B			
Periodic acid-Schiff			
Terminal deoxynucleotidyl transferase			

19. Match the findings with the most appropriate disorder. The disorders may be used more than once, but each finding should be associated with only one disorder.

A. _____ Marked toxic vacuoles

B. _____ Marked toxic granulation

C. _____ Marked eosinophilia

D. _____ Marked basophilia

E. _____ Philadelphia chromosome

F. _____ Frequent Döhle bodies

G. _____ Elevated LAP

a. Leukemoid reaction

b. CML

20. Interpret the laboratory data in the following chart, and match each patient with one of the following myelodysplastic syndromes. Each syndrome may be used only once.

a. Refractory anemia
b. Refractory anemia with ringed sideroblasts
c. Refractory anemia with excess blasts
d. Refractory anemia with excess blasts in transformation
e. Chronic myelomonocytic leukemia

Laboratory Test	Patient A	Patient B	Patient C	Patient D	Patient E
Platelet count	↓	↓	↓	Normal	Normal
RBC count	↓	↓	↓	↓	↓ (Dimorphic)
WBC count	↓	↑ with monocytosis	↓	↓	Normal
% Blasts in peripheral blood	1	4	6	0	0
% Blasts in bone marrow	15	15	25 with Auer rods	3	4
% Ringed sideroblasts in bone marrow	10	9	2	7	25
Chromosomal abnormality	5q⁻	12q⁻	5q⁻	5q⁻	5q⁻
Interpretation					

21. Match the FAB classification on the left with the appropriate acute lymphoblastic leukemia characteristic on the right. Each answer may be used only once.

A. _____ L1

B. _____ L2

C. _____ L3

a. Burkitt's type

b. Small, uniform lymphoblasts; seen most often in children

c. Large, pleomorphic lymphoblasts; seen most often in adults

22. Label the following protein electrophoretic densitometer tracing.

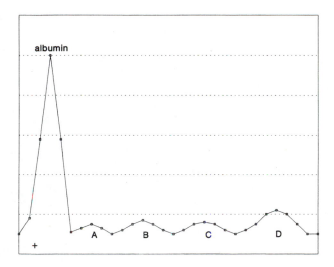

A.

B.

C.

D.

23. Identify the following protein electrophoretic densitometer tracings.

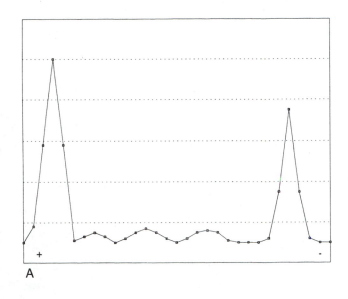

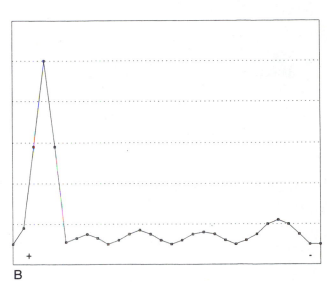

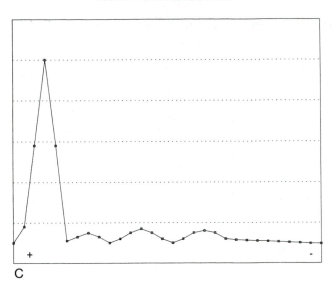

A.

B.

C.

24. Define the following:
   A. Monoclonal gammopathy

   B. Rouleaux

   C. Serum protein electrophoresis

D. Macroglobulinemia

E. Cryoglobulin

25. Label the anatomic compartments of the lymph node.

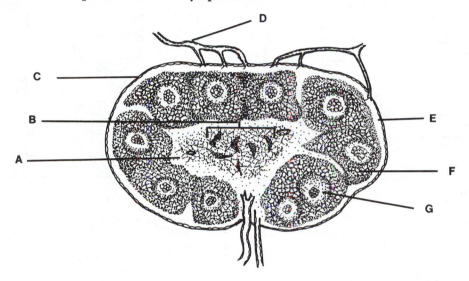

A.

B.

C.

D.

E.

F.

G.

26. Interpret the following laboratory data and give the most probable diagnosis. Your choices are any of the acute myeloid leukemias (M1 through M6) and any of the acute lymphoblastic leukemias (L1 through L3).

Laboratory Test	Normal Range	Patient A	Patient B	Patient C
Patient data		33-year-old male with slight splenomegaly and bleeding of 2 weeks duration	55-year-old female with fatigue for 3–4 months	4-year-old male with multiple bruises
WBC (×10⁹/L)	4.4–10.8	32.1	4.3	13.6
Hemoglobin (g/L)	Male: 135–180 Female: 120–160	95	80	115
Platelet count (×10⁹/L)	140–415	25	85	42
WBC Differential % Blasts	0	80	3	92
% Promyelocytes	0	15	1	0
% Myelocytes	0	0	0	0
% Metamyelocytes	0	0	0	0
% Band neutrophils	2–5	0	3	0
% Segmented neutrophils	48–70	1	20	3
% Lymphocytes	18–54	4	69	5
% Monocytes	2–10	0	4	0
Comments on peripheral blood film	Normocytic, normochromic	Schistocytes and faggots of Auer rods noted	12 NRBCs pseudo-Pelger cells seen	Normocytic, normochromic
Comments on bone marrow preparation	Normocellular	Myeloid hyperplasia	Marked erythroid hyperplasia and ringed sideroblasts	Marked hyperplasia
Peroxidase stain	−	+	−	−
Specific esterase stain	−	+	−	−
Non-specific esterase stain	−	−	−	−
Periodic acid-Schiff stain	−	Weakly +	+	Weakly +
TdT	−	−	−	+
CD 14	−	−	−	−
CD 10 (CALLA)	−	−	−	+/−
CD 19	−	−	−	+
HLA-DR	−	−	−	+
Interpretation				

27. Match the findings with the most appropriate disorder. The disorders may be used more than once, but each finding should be associated with only one disorder.

A. _____ Philadelphia chromosome

B. _____ Sternal tenderness

C. _____ Left shift

D. _____ Autoimmune phenomenon

E. _____ Elevated uric acid, LDH, and B$_{12}$ levels

F. _____ Decreased LAP

a. CLL

b. CML

Answers to Section Two Worksheets

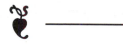

1. Cells counted = 475
   Dilution = 1 : 20, therefore the reciprocal is 20
   Area = $1 \times 1 \times 4 = 4$, therefore the reciprocal is ¼ or 0.25
   Depth = 1/10, therefore the reciprocal is 10

   Actual cell count = (475)(10)(0.25)(10)
   $$= 23.8 \times 10^3/mm^3 \text{ or } 23.8 \times 10^9/L$$
   REF: H:527–528; L:322; M:x; T:345–347

2. A. Cells counted = 53
      Dilution = 1 : 10, therefore the reciprocal is 10
      Area = $1 \times 1 \times 9 = 9$, therefore the reciprocal is 1/9 or 0.11
      Depth = 1/10, therefore the reciprocal is 10

      Actual cell count = (53)(10)(0.11)(10)
      $$= 589/mm^3 \text{ or } 0.589 \times 10^9/L$$

   B. WBC = $10.0 \times 10^9/L$
      Relative eosinophil count from the differential = 6%
      Absolute eosinophil count = $6\% \times (10.0 \times 10^9/L)$
      $$= 0.06 \times (10.0 \times 10^9/L)$$
      $$= 0.600 \times 10^9/L$$

   C. Reported
   REF: H:529–530; L:329–331; M:x; T:337–338

3. Corrected WBC $= \dfrac{(21.0 \times 10^9/L) \times 100}{20 + 100} = 17.5 \times 10^9/L$
   REF: H:547; L:328; M:x; T:347

4. A. Relative neutrophil count = segmented neutrophils + band neutrophils
      $$= 80\% + 5\% = 85\%$$
      Absolute neutrophil count = $85\% \times (15.0 \times 10^9/L)$
      $$= 0.85 \times (15.0 \times 10^9/L) = 12.8 \times 10^9/L$$
      REF: H:530; L:328; M:52; T:137

   B. Relative neutrophilia; absolute neutrophilia. REF: H:243, 245; L:328; M:52; T:144–145

   C. Absolute lymphocyte count = $13\% \times (15.0 \times 10^9/L)$
      $$= 0.13 \times (15.0 \times 10^9/L) = 2.0 \times 10^9/L$$
      REF: H:530; L:328; M:52; T:168

   D. Relative lymphopenia; absolute-normal. REF: H:x; L:328; M:52; T:168

E. Absolute monocyte count $= 1\% \times (15.0 \times 10^9/L)$
$$= 0.01 \times (15.0 \times 10^9/L) = 0.2 \times 10^9/L$$
REF: H:530; L:328; M:52; T:137

F. Relative monocytopenia; absolute-normal. REF: H:x; L:328; M:52; T:144–145

G. Absolute eosinophil count $= 1\% \times (15.0 \times 10^9/L)$
$$= 0.01 \times (15.0 \times 10^9/L) = 0.2 \times 10^9/L$$
REF: H:530; L:328; M:52; T:137

H. Relative-normal; absolute-normal. REF: H:x; L:328; M:52; T:144–145

5. A. Lymphocytes
   B. Mononuclear cells
   C. Granulocytes
   REF: H:555; L:498; M:x; T:312

6. A. Monocytes
   B. Neutrophils
   C. Eosinophils
   D. Lymphocytes
   REF: H:558; L:523; M:x; T:x

7. A. Monocytes
   B. Lymphocytes
   C. Platelet debris
   D. Neutrophils
   E. Eosinophils
   REF: H:559; L:506; M:x; T:319

8. A. Basophils
   B. Mononuclear WBCs
   C. Polymorphonuclear WBCs
   REF: H:559; L:507; M:x; T:320

9. A. Substances that stimulate the proliferation and differentiation of stem cells. REF: H:242; L:50; M:56; T:129
   B. Neutrophils that adhere to the endothelial lining of blood vessels. REF: H:242; L:294; M:55; T:130
   C. An increased percentage of immature neutrophils. REF: H:243; L:338; M:253; T:137
   D. Primary granules in the cytoplasm of neutrophils. REF: H:243; L:339; M:258; T:145
   E. Large, bluish structures in the cytoplasm of leukocytes. REF: H:243; L:339; M:258; T:146
   F. The act of ingesting and degrading particles. REF: H:244; L:296; M:58; T:134
   G. A decreased number of neutrophils in the peripheral blood. REF: H:245; L:337; M:255; T:145

10. A. b. REF: H:247; L:337; M:257; T:145
    B. c. REF: H:249; L:358; M:260; T:146
    C. f. REF: H:252; L:357; M:260; T:146
    D. d. REF: H:252; L:356; M:259; T:146
    E. h. REF: H:250; L:359; M:260; T:147
    F. a. REF: H:243; L:338–339; M:252, 258; T:137, 144–145
    G. e. REF: H:252; L:357; M:259; T:146

11. Myeloblast, promyelocyte, myelocyte, metamyelocyte, band neutrophil, segmented neutrophil. REF: H:30–32; L:292–294; M:53; T:131

12. A. Metamyelocyte. REF: H:31; L:393; M:54; T:131–132

   B. Lymphocyte. REF: H:35–36; L:291; M:67; T:157

   C. Eosinophil. REF: H:33; L:290; M:Plate II-G; T:Plate 33

   D. Myeloblast. REF: H:30–31; L:292–293; M:53; T:131

   E. Variant lymphocyte. REF: H:36; L:291; M:68; T:158

   F. Monocyte. REF: H:34–35; L:291; M:62; T:133

   G. Plasma cell. REF: H:36–37; L:311; M:73; T:163

13. A. b

   B. c

   C. a

   REF: H:404–407; L:360; M:265; T:147

14. A. Phagocytosis of bacteria and other foreign organisms. REF: H:244; L:296; M:57; T:134

   B. Limit allergic reactions and digests parasites. REF: H:x; L:298; M:60; T:136

   C. Release histamine during allergic reactions. REF: H:34; L:299; M:61; T:136

   D. Ingest foreign substances, processes antigens for immune response, and phagocytizes dying cells. REF: H:35; L:301; M:64; T:136

   E. Responds to foreign antigens with cellular and humoral immunity. REF: H:260; L:308; M:65; T:158

   F. Produce antibody to foreign antigens. REF: H:37; L:308; M:73; T:162

15. A. e

   B. a

   C. d

   REF: H:262–263; L:352–353; M:267–270; T:168–174

16. IgA, IgD, IgE, IgG, IgM. REF: H:367; L:475; M:73; T:x

17. A. g

   B. f

   C. e

   D. d

   E. c

   F. a

   G. b

   REF: H:277; L:422–426; M:330–336; T:195

18.

Leukocyte Special Stains			
Special Stains	Constituent Stained	Cell Type Stained	Results/ Comments
Leukocyte alkaline phosphatase (LAP)	Enzyme: LAP	Neutrophils	Increased in pregnancy, polycythemia vera, infections, leukemoid reaction, and CML blast crisis. Decreased in CML, PNH, sideroblastic anemia, secondary polycythemia, and sickle cell anemia
Myeloperoxidase	Enzyme: Peroxidase	Myeloid cells	Increased in AML, AMoL, and AMMoL
Specific esterase (naphthol AS-D chloroacetate	Enzyme: Esterase	Granulocytes, granulocytic precursors, and mast cells	Increased in AML, AMMoL, and mast cell disease
Non-specific esterase (alpha-naphthyl butyrate)	Enzyme: Esterase	Megakaryocytes, monocytes, monocytic precursors, granulocytes, macrophages, and histiocytes	Increased in ALL, AML, AMoL, AMMoL, and CMMoL
Combined esterase	Enzyme: Esterase	Monocytes, granulocytes, histiocytes, macrophages, and mesothelial	Increased in AMoL and AMMoL
Tartrate-resistant acid phosphatase (TRAP)	Enzyme: Acid phosphatase	Hairy cells and histiocytes	Increased in hairy cell leukemia, Sézary syndrome, and prolymphocytic leukemia
Sudan black B	Lipids	Granulocytes, monocytes, promyelocytes, and myeloblasts	Increased in AML, AMoL, and AMMoL
Periodic acid-Schiff	Glycogen	Granulocytes, monocytes, megakaryocytes, and M6 erythrocytes	Increased in ALL, AMoL, AMMoL, erythroleukemia, and Ewing's sarcoma
Terminal deoxynucleotidyl transferase	DNA polymerase	Early lymphocytes	Increased in T-cell and precursor B-cell ALL, AML, CML, and lymphoma

REF: H:569–578; L:380–387; M:318–320, 328, 342; T:199, 201–205, 228–229

19. A. a
    B. a
    C. b
    D. b
    E. b
    F. a
    G. a
    REF: H:332; L:437; M:284; T:228–229

20. A. c
    B. e
    C. d
    D. a
    E. b
    REF: H:295–300; L:412–414; M:305–308; T:249–251

21. A. b
    B. c
    C. a
    REF: H:283; L:450; M:339; T:195

22. A. Alpha 1
    B. Alpha 2
    C. Beta
    D. Gamma
    REF: H:371; L:476; M:x; T:218

23. A. IgG myeloma with a gamma spike
    B. Normal
    C. Hypogammaglobulinemia
    REF: H:371; L:476; M:x; T:218

24. A. Plasma cell disorders that produce a single class of antibody and show a spike in one region on protein electrophoresis. REF: H:367, 371; L:474–475; M:x; T:x
    B. Arrangements of RBCs that resemble stacks of coins. REF: H:369; L:89; M:99; T:93
    C. Analysis of serum proteins based on the movement of different sized molecules through an electrical field. REF: H:370; L:475; M:x; T:218
    D. An increased concentration of monoclonal IgM. REF: H:379; L:478; M:362; T:218
    E. A protein that precipitates at low temperatures. REF: H:379; L:x; M:x; T:219

25. A. Paracortex
    B. Medulla
    C. Capsule
    D. Lymphatic vessels
    E. Sinus
    F. Cortex
    G. Germinal/follicular center
    REF: H:393; L:307; M:16; T:156

26. A. M3. REF: H:280; L:424; M:332–333; T:196

    B. M6. REF: H:281; L:426; M:319–320, 335–336; T:197, 205

    C. L1. REF: H:282–288; L:389, 450; M:339, 342; T:198–200

27. A. b. REF: H:326; L:435; M:279; T:227

    B. b. REF: H:329; L:435; M:280; T:227

    C. b. REF: H:329; L:435; M:281; T:228

    D. a. REF: H:313; L:457; M:358; T:213

    E. b. REF: H:330; L:x; M:281; T:x

    F. b. REF: H:326; L:436; M:281; T:228

Section Two Questions

Select the Best Answer	Answers & References

1. Cerebrospinal fluid is pipetted to the 1.0 mark of the WBC pipet, and the number of cells counted in the nine primary squares on both sides equals 200 WBCs. The WBC count is _____ $\times 10^9$/L.
  A. 1.1
  B. 2.2
  C. 28
  D. 360
	A
	H:528−529
	L:322
	M:x
	T:345−347

2. A differential leukocyte count revealed 225 nucleated RBCs/100 WBCs. The total leukocyte count was 7.0×10^9/L. The corrected total leukocyte count is _____ $\times 10^9$/L.
  A. 2.2
  B. 3.1
  C. 4.6
  D. 7.2
	C
	H:547
	L:328
	M:x
	T:347

3. A patient has a WBC count of 7.5×10^9/L with 55% neutrophils. The absolute neutrophil count ($\times 10^9$/L) and the appropriate terminology are:
  A. 3.4, relative neutropenia, absolute-normal.
  B. 3.4, relative-normal, absolute neutrophilia.
  C. 4.1, relative neutrophilia, absolute neutropenia.
  D. 4.1, relative-normal, absolute-normal.
	D
	H:530
	L:328
	M:52
	T:137, 144−145

4. Granulopoiesis is dependent on the presence of growth-promoting substances called:
  A. Colony-stimulating factors.
  B. Growth hormone.
  C. Cell substance factors.
  D. Stem cell factors.
	A
	H:242
	L:50
	M:56
	T:129

5. Which of the following is *not* true?
  A. Neutrophils exchange freely between marginating and circulating pools.
  B. The circulating half-life of neutrophils is approximately 7−10 hours.
  C. Neutrophils exchange freely between blood and tissues.
  D. Neutrophils can be held in the marrow for future release into the peripheral blood.
	C
	H:242
	L:294−295
	M:55
	T:x

Select the Best Answer	Answers & References
6. The term "left shift" refers to:	A
A. Immature granulocytes.	H:243
B. Immature lymphocytes.	L:338
C. Immature monocytes.	M:253
D. Leukocytosis.	T:137
7. A left shift is most likely to occur in:	A
A. Bacterial infections.	H:243
B. Viral infections.	L:337
C. Parasitic infections.	M:252–253
D. All infections.	T:x
8. In a normal healthy adult, how does the neutrophil count vary?	B
A. It is higher during the day than at night.	H:243
B. It is higher at night than during the day.	L:x
C. It is constant.	M:55
D. It varies unpredictably.	T:134
9. Qualitative or morphologic changes which may occur in neutrophils include all the following *except*:	C
A. Döhle bodies.	H:243
B. Toxic granulation.	L:338
C. Howell-Jolly bodies.	M:98
D. Cytoplasmic vacuoles.	T:50, 145–146
10. The neutrophil locomotion process is stimulated by:	D
A. Sodium.	H:244
B. Chloride.	L:297
C. Manganese.	M:57
D. Chemotactic factors.	T:134
11. Proteins, such as antibody and complement, that aid phagocytosis of microorganisms are called:	B
A. Lysosomes.	H:244
B. Opsonins.	L:297
C. Vesicles.	M:64
D. Lipoproteins.	T:135
12. During phagocytosis, neutrophils metabolize glucose by:	B
A. Aerobic glycolysis to provide ATP.	H:245
B. Anaerobic glycolysis to provide ATP.	L:295
C. Neoglycogenesis to produce oxygen.	M:58
D. Neoglycogenesis to produce hydrogen oxygenase.	T:134

Select the Best Answer	Answers & References
13. Which of the following is *not* a mechanism by which neutropenia may be produced? A. Decreased production by the bone marrow B. Impaired release from the tissues to the blood C. Increased destruction D. Maldistribution between marginating and circulating pools	B H:246 L:337–338 M:56 T:145
14. Hyposegmentation is characteristic of the _____ anomaly. A. Alder-Reilly B. May-Hegglin C. Pelger-Huët D. Job's	C H:252 L:356 M:259 T:146
15. Blue-staining cytoplasmic inclusions that resemble Döhle bodies may be seen in the _____ anomaly. A. Alder-Reilly B. May-Hegglin C. Pelger-Huët D. Job's	 B H:252 L:357 M:260 T:146
16. Hypersegmentation of neutrophils is defined as more than _____ segments. A. Three B. Five C. Seven D. Nine	 B H:252 L:357 M:168 T:146
17. Proteins that work in concert with colony-stimulating factors as well as enhance production and maturation of WBC stem cells are called: A. Erythropoietins. B. Thrombopoietins. C. Interleukins. D. Burst-forming units.	C H:27 L:177 M:64 T:45
18. The granulocytic cells capable of mitosis are: A. Uncommitted stem cell, committed stem cell, and myeloblast. B. Myeloblast, promyelocyte, myelocyte, and band neutrophil. C. Committed stem cell, myeloblast, promyelocyte, and myelocyte. D. Metamyelocyte, band neutrophil, and segmented neutrophil.	C H:30 L:293 M:54 T:129
19. The marginating pool of neutrophils is located: A. On the walls of the blood vessels. B. In the spleen. C. Next to the marrow sinuses. D. In the tissues.	A H:30 L:295 M:x T:130

Select the Best Answer	Answers & References
20. The cellular structure(s) that differentiates the promyelocyte from the myeloblast is (are) the: A. Golgi body. B. Indented nucleus. C. Secondary granules. D. Primary granules.	D H:31 L:293 M:53 T:131
21. The cellular structure(s) that differentiates the band neutrophil from the metamyelocyte is (are) the: A. Secondary granules. B. Horseshoe-shaped nucleus. C. Nucleolus. D. Primary granules.	B H:31 L:294 M:74 T:131–132
22. The beginning of neutrophilic differentiation begins at what stage? A. Promyelocyte B. Myelocyte C. Metamyelocyte D. Band neutrophil	B H:31 L:293 M:x T:131
23. Tissue basophils are also known as _____ cells. A. Mott B. Plasma C. Mast D. Turk	C H:34 L:299 M:x T:132
24. Which of the following are most closely associated with Gaucher's disease? A. Splenomegaly, Gaucher's cells in bone marrow, and elevated serum acid phosphatase B. Splenomegaly, Gaucher's cells in bone marrow, and elevated serum alkaline phosphatase C. Hepatosplenomegaly, Gaucher's cells in bone marrow, and elevated serum acid phosphatase D. Hepatomegaly, Gaucher's cells in bone marrow, and elevated serum alkaline phosphatase	C H:404 L:x M:264 T:x
25. Patients with mucopolysaccharidoses may exhibit which of the following in their peripheral blood? A. Alder-Reilly bodies B. Auer rods C. Heinz bodies D. Howell-Jolly bodies	A H:408 L:360 M:259 T:146

Select the Best Answer	Answers & References

26. The condition most closely associated with Niemann-Pick disease is a(an):
    A. Deficiency of sphingomyelinase.
    B. Deficiency of sulfaminidase.
    C. Excess of sulfaminidase.
    D. Excess of sphingomyelinase.
	A
	H:406
	L:360
	M:265
	T:147

27. What is the circulating form of macrophages?
    A. Segmented neutrophils
    B. Lymphocytes
    C. Rubricytes
    D. Monocytes
	D
	H:35
	L:300
	M:62
	T:139

28. The function of the T lymphocyte is to:
    A. Produce immune globulins.
    B. Interact with antibody to destroy antibody-coated targets.
    C. Phagocytize bacteria and cellular debris.
    D. Participate in cellular immunity.
	D
	H:24
	L:308
	M:69
	T:158

29. T lymphocytes are cells that differentiate in the:
    A. Thyroid.
    B. Tonsils.
    C. Tongue.
    D. Thymus.
	D
	H:35
	L:305
	M:69
	T:161

30. B lymphocytes are cells that differentiate in the:
    A. Bone marrow.
    B. Bursa of Fabricius.
    C. Brain.
    D. Basement membrane.
	A
	H:35
	L:304
	M:70
	T:154

31. Plasma cells originate from:
    A. B lymphocytes.
    B. T lymphocytes.
    C. Monocytes.
    D. Macrophages.
	A
	H:36
	L:308
	M:72
	T:162

32. Stimulated, atypical, and reactive lymphocytes refer to _____ lymphocytes.
    A. Benign
    B. Malignant
    C. Variant
    D. Viral
	C
	H:258
	L:348–349
	M:68
	T:157–158

Select the Best Answer	Answers & References

33. Which of the following is most consistent with the cytologic findings of a reactive lymphocyte?
  A. Densely stained, clumped chromatin and scant, blue, vacuolated cytoplasm
  B. Finely to coarsely clumped chromatin, frequently with nucleoli and abundant, blue, vacuolated cytoplasm scalloping around adjacent RBCs
  C. Lightly stained chromatin with a lacy appearance and abundant gray cytoplasm which remains rigid when touching adjacent RBCs
  D. Clumped chromatin with scant gray cytoplasm
	B
	H:259
	L:349–350
	M:68
	T:158

34. The population with the highest susceptibility to infectious mononucleosis is:
  A. Middle-class teenagers and young adults.
  B. Lower socioeconomic adults.
  C. Lower socioeconomic children and teenagers.
  D. Affluent children.
	A
	H:261
	L:351
	M:267
	T:170

35. Which of the following is *not* included in the classical description of infectious mononucleosis?
  A. Sore throat, fever, and swollen cervical lymph nodes
  B. Left shift
  C. Absolute lymphocytosis
  D. ≥10% variant lymphocytes
	B
	H:261
	L:351–352
	M:268
	T:170

36. Criteria for the diagnosis of infectious mononucleosis are:
  A. Negative heterophile antibody test and CMV antibody titer.
  B. Positive heterophile antibody test or EBV antibody titer.
  C. Positive heterophile antibody test or HIV antibody titer.
  D. Positive heterophile antibody test or CMV titer.
	B
	H:261
	L:352
	M:268–270
	T:170

37. The cell marker used to identify mature B-cells is:
  A. T4 antigens.
  B. T8 antigens.
  C. Cytoplasmic immunoglobulin.
  D. Surface immunoglobulin.
	D
	H:285
	L:x
	M:71
	T:160

38. Pre-B and plasma cells are identified by:
  A. T4 antigens.
  B. T8 antigens.
  C. Cytoplasmic immunoglobulin.
  D. Surface immunoglobulin.
	C
	H:285
	L:x
	M:71
	T:160

Select the Best Answer	Answers & References

39. If a patient presents with signs and symptoms consistent with infectious mononucleosis but the heterophile antibody titer is negative, the next diagnostic step would be to:
  A. Immediately repeat the heterophile antibody test.
  B. Immediately repeat the CBC.
  C. Repeat the heterophile antibody test after 1 week.
  D. Perform a CMV-IgM antibody test.
	C
	H:262
	L:352
	M:x
	T:x

40. Antigens which identify lymphocytes as helper cells develop from _____ lymphocytes and are known as _____ .
  A. B, CD4
  B. B, CD8
  C. T, CD4
  D. T, CD8
	C
	H:367
	L:x
	M:x
	T:161

41. The cells that produce immunoglobulins are:
  A. B lymphocytes.
  B. T lymphocytes.
  C. B & T lymphocytes.
  D. All lymphocytes.
	A
	H:368
	L:308
	M:73
	T:158

42. Russell bodies are:
  A. Multinucleated plasma cells.
  B. Aggregates of immunoglobulins.
  C. Tumor masses.
  D. Lytic bone lesions.
	B
	H:375
	L:477
	M:73
	T:163

43. The most numerous cell type in the marrow throughout infancy is the:
  A. Erythrocyte.
  B. Granulocyte.
  C. Lymphocyte.
  D. Monocyte.
	C
	H:242
	L:x
	M:4
	T:x

44. The majority of total immunoglobulin in healthy patients is attributed to:
  A. IgA.
  B. IgD.
  C. IgG.
  D. IgM.
	C
	H:370
	L:475
	M:75
	T:x

45. Which of the following is *not* a major type of leukocyte found in peripheral blood?
  A. Granulocyte
  B. Lymphocyte
  C. Monocyte
  D. Histiocyte
	D
	H:241
	L:289
	M:52
	T:129

Select the Best Answer	Answers & References

46. The cytologic peculiarities of the Alder-Reilly anomaly may be found in:
  A. Granulocytes.
  B. Lymphocytes.
  C. Granulocytes and lymphocytes.
  D. Granulocytes, lymphocytes, and monocytes.
	D
	H:252
	L:357
	M:259
	T:146

47. Which of the following environmental factors does *not* appear to influence one's predisposition for leukemia?
  A. Ionizing exposure
  B. Bacterial infections
  C. Toxic chemical exposure
  D. Viral infections
	B
	H:268–269
	L:408
	M:313–314
	T:187

48. Acute leukemias primarily affect:
  A. Children, progress rapidly, and have mature cells in the peripheral circulation.
  B. All ages, progress rapidly, and have immature cells in the peripheral circulation.
  C. Young adults, progress slowly, and have immature cells in the peripheral circulation.
  D. Adults, progress slowly, and have mature cells in the peripheral circulation.
	B
	H:269
	L:408–409
	M:315
	T:190

49. Chronic leukemias primarily affect:
  A. Children, progress rapidly, and have mature cells in the peripheral circulation.
  B. All ages, progress rapidly, and have immature cells in the peripheral circulation.
  C. Young adults, progress slowly, and have immature cells in the peripheral circulation.
  D. Adults, progress slowly, and have mature cells in the peripheral circulation.
	D
	H:269
	L:408–409
	M:315
	T:226–228

50. The commonly used classification system for leukemias is the:
  A. CD.
  B. CSL.
  C. M.
  D. FAB.
	D
	H:277
	L:409
	M:329
	T:194

51. The peak incidence of acute myeloblastic leukemia occurs in:
  A. Infants.
  B. Children.
  C. Adults.
  D. Geriatric patients.
	C
	H:269
	L:422
	M:327
	T:195–196

Select the Best Answer	Answers & References

52. Myeloperoxidase is *not* exhibited in:
    A. Neutrophils.
    B. Basophils.
    C. Lymphocytes.
    D. Monocytes.
	C
	H:273
	L:x
	M:317
	T:202

53. A positive periodic acid-Schiff reaction would favor a diagnosis of:
    A. M1.
    B. M2.
    C. M4.
    D. M6.
	D
	H:274
	L:421
	M:328
	T:205

54. The stain(s) used to differentiate AML from ALL is (are):
    A. Myeloperoxidase.
    B. Sudan black B.
    C. Myeloperoxidase and Sudan black B.
    D. Sudan black B and periodic acid-Schiff.
	C
	H:274
	L:386–389
	M:318
	T:201–202

55. The Philadelphia chromosome is most often associated with:
    A. AML.
    B. ALL.
    C. CML.
    D. CLL.
	C
	H:276
	L:435
	M:281
	T:227

56. The most frequent chromosomal abnormality in the myelodysplastic syndromes (MDSs) is:
    A. 1.
    B. 5.
    C. 10.
    D. 15.
	B
	H:294
	L:417
	M:x
	T:258

57. The MDS which most frequently transforms into ANLL is:
    A. Refractory anemia with excess blasts.
    B. Refractory anemia with excess blasts in transformation.
    C. Refractory anemia with ringed sideroblasts.
    D. Chronic myelomonocytic leukemia.
	B
	H:299
	L:x
	M:307
	T:253

58. A gene that may produce neoplastic transformation is called a(n):
    A. Protogene.
    B. Pregene.
    C. Oncogene.
    D. Autogene.
	C
	H:328
	L:420
	M:x
	T:187

Select the Best Answer	Answers & References
59. A patient who has persistent leukocytosis, Döhle bodies, and an elevated LAP score most likely has:	C
A. Chronic myelogenous leukemia.	H:332
B. Chronic lymphocytic leukemia.	L:437
C. Leukemoid reaction.	M:284
D. Pelger-Huët anomaly.	T:228
60. The disease most frequently confused with idiopathic myelofibrosis is:	A
A. Chronic myelogenous leukemia.	H:345
B. Acute myelogenous leukemia.	L:439
C. Sarcoidosis.	M:289
D. Metastatic carcinoma.	T:228
61. Which of the following laboratory tests may require additional calculations for polycythemia vera patients?	B
A. CBC	H:350
B. PT/APTT	L:608–609
C. Uric acid	M:407
D. Vitamin B_{12}	T:384
62. Which of the following is most important in diagnosing polycythemia?	A
A. Elevated RBC mass	H:351
B. Elevated hematocrit	L:433–434
C. Elevated hemoglobin	M:295
D. Elevated RBC count	T:231
63. The primary treatment(s) in polycythemia vera is (are):	D
A. Anticoagulation therapy.	H:353
B. Splenectomy and phlebotomy.	L:434
C. Chemotherapy and splenectomy.	M:292
D. Phlebotomy and chemotherapy.	T:232
64. The most common type of leukemia is:	B
A. CML.	H:312
B. CLL.	L:455
C. AML.	M:x
D. ALL.	T:213
65. Terminal deoxynucleotidyl transferase is an enzyme that is present in:	A
A. Immature lymphocytes.	H:276
B. Immature monocytes.	L:389
C. Mature lymphocytes.	M:342
D. Mature monocytes.	T:199

Select the Best Answer	Answers & References

66. Which of the following occurs most frequently in the pediatric age group?
   A. L1
   B. L2
   C. L3
   D. L4
	A
	H:287
	L:450
	M:339
	T:198

67. Which of the following occurs most frequently in the adult age group?
   A. L1
   B. L2
   C. L3
   D. L4
	B
	H:287
	L:450
	M:339
	T:198

68. Smudge cells are frequently evident in:
   A. CLL.
   B. CML.
   C. ALL.
   D. AML.
	A
	H:312
	L:456
	M:358
	T:214

69. In a case of suspected CLL, a positive tartrate-resistant acid phosphatase stain would indicate that the most likely diagnosis is:
   A. B-CLL.
   B. T-CLL.
   C. Sézary syndrome.
   D. Hairy cell leukemia.
	D
	H:323
	L:384
	M:215
	T:215

70. Malignant plasma cell disorders are often called _____ gammopathies.
   A. Aclonal
   B. Hypoclonal
   C. Monoclonal
   D. Polyclonal
	C
	H:367
	L:474
	M:360–362
	T:217

71. A common hematologic manifestation of multiple myeloma is:
   A. Rouleaux.
   B. Red background on Wright's-stained smears.
   C. Elevated neutrophil count.
   D. Circulating megakaryocytes.
	A
	H:369
	L:477
	M:361
	T:217

72. Which of the following does *not* result from the malignant proliferation of plasma cells?
   A. Lytic bone lesions
   B. Pancytopenia
   C. Increased amount of normal immunoglobulins
   D. Production of abnormal immunoglobulins
	C
	H:376
	L:476–477
	M:360
	T:217–218

Select the Best Answer	Answers & References
73. The most diagnostic cell type seen in Waldenström's macroglobulinemia is the: A. Mature lymphocyte. B. Early plasma cell. C. Plasmacytoid lymphocyte. D. Mature monocyte.	C H:379 L:478 M:362 T:218–219
74. Bleeding problems in Waldenström's macroglobulinemia are caused by: A. Hypovolemia. B. Thrombocytosis. C. Splenomegaly. D. IgM-coated platelets.	D H:379 L:478 M:362 T:x
75. The absence of a peak after the beta peak in a serum protein electrophoresis densitometer tracing is consistent with: A. Polyclonal hypergammaglobulinemia. B. Waldenström's macroglobulinemia. C. Multiple myeloma. D. Hypogammaglobulinemia.	D H:371 L:476 M:x T:218
76. Which of the following most likely indicates Waldenström's macroglobulinemia instead of multiple myeloma? A. Significant organomegaly and hyperviscosity B. Significant hyperviscosity and lytic bone lesions C. Significant organomegaly and lytic bone lesions D. Significant hyperviscosity and renal failure	A H:379 L:476–478 M:360–362 T:217–219
77. An elevated PT and APTT in a patient with Waldenström's macroglobulinemia is most likely due to: A. Warfarin therapy. B. Heparin therapy. C. Aspirin ingestion. D. IgM interference.	D H:380 L:478 M:362 T:x
78. The diagnostic cell in Hodgkin's disease is the: A. Reactive lymphoblast. B. Non-cleaved lymphoblast. C. Reilly-Stanokovich cell. D. Reed-Sternberg cell.	D H:385 L:463 M:347 T:219
79. One of the more common childhood non-Hodgkin's lymphomas in the United States is: A. Carmen's. B. Burkitt's. C. Sézary's. D. Rapaport's.	B H:397 L:x M:355 T:x

Select the Best Answer	Answers & References
80. The peak incidence of acute lymphoblastic leukemia occurs in:	B
A. Infants.	H:269
B. Children.	L:448
C. Adults.	M:337
D. Geriatric patients.	T:198
81. Which of the following would indicate ALL instead of AML?	B
A. Auer rods	H:270
B. A positive TdT stain	L:389
C. A positive peroxidase stain	M:342
D. A positive Sudan black B stain	T:199

Section Three

HEMOSTASIS

Objectives for
Hemostasis Section

After studying the referenced material for each hemostasis chapter outline, completing the worksheet, and taking the section test, the student will be able to:

1 Identify general component parts of blood vessels

2 List hemostatic substances produced by the endothelium and discuss the role of each substance in hemostasis

3 Define ecchymoses, petechiae, purpura, telangiectasia, and spontaneous bleeds

4 Select appropriate coagulation tests to aid in differentiating hemostatic disorders

5 Interpret clinical and laboratory data to identify common coagulation disorders

6 Differentiate between the maturational stages of the megakaryocytic cell line

7 Calculate manual platelet counts, international normalized ratio, and anticoagulant to blood ratio adjustments

8 Describe the structure of a platelet

9 Identify the steps in platelet kinetics

10 Compare and contrast reactive thrombocytosis and thrombocytosis caused by myeloproliferative disorders

11 Define thrombocytopenia, thrombocytosis, and thrombocytopathy

12 Explain how aspirin ingestion interferes with platelet function

13 List the coagulation factors by Roman numerals and common names

14 Specify common characteristics of the fibrinogen family, prothrombin family, and contact family

15 Illustrate the interaction of the coagulation factors with one another, with their regulators, and with the fibrinolytic pathway

16 Discuss the mode of action and monitoring of therapeutic anticoagulants

17 Use substitution studies to identify a coagulation factor deficiency

18 Explain the fibrinolytic mechanism

19 Compare and contrast primary and secondary fibrinolysis

20 State the purpose of the following laboratory tests:

Activated partial thromboplastin time	Platelet aggregation studies
Activated whole blood clotting time	Platelet count
Antiplatelet antibodies	Platelet factor 3 availability
Aspirin tolerance test	Platelet neutralization procedure
Bleeding time	Platelet retention studies
Clot retraction	Protamine sulfate test
D-Dimer assay	Prothrombin time
Euglobulin lysis time	Stypven time
Factor assay	Substitution studies
Fibrin(ogen) split products assay	Thrombin time
Fibrinopeptides assay	Tourniquet test
Fibrinogen assay	Urea solubility test
Lee-White whole blood clotting time	Whole blood clot lysis
Plasminogen assay	

Chapter 13

The Vascular Component, Platelets, and Related Disorders

I. The vascular system: Arteries, veins, and capillaries

A. Vessel structure: Blood vessels vary in thickness of the following layers, but the components' functions remain the same.

1. Endothelial cells: The innermost layer of the vessels is antithrombotic and manufactures substances necessary for hemostasis. These substances include the following:

   a. ADPase: Degrades ADP (adenosine diphosphate)

   b. Collagen: Activates coagulation factors and stimulates platelet adhesion

   c. Glycocalyx: Coats the endothelial surface with heparan sulfate

   d. Prostacyclin: Dilates vessels and inhibits platelet aggregation

   e. Thrombomodulin: Neutralizes thrombin and enhances protein C activity

   f. Tissue plasminogen activator (tPA): Assists in clot lysis

   g. von Willebrand's factor: Regulates platelet adhesion

2. Subendothelial cells: A middle layer of the vessels acts as a thrombogenic agent.

3. Basement membrane: A middle layer of the vessels provides a matrix for subendothelial and endothelial cells.

4. Collagen and elastic fibers: The outermost layer of the vessels controls vessel dilation and constriction. Platelet adhesion and aggregation are also promoted by this layer.

B. Clinical evidence of dysfunction.

1. Ecchymoses: Large venous hemorrhages into subcutaneous tissue

2. Petechiae: Minute hemorrhages from small vessels

3. Purpura: A general term for bleeding from capillaries into the skin and mucosa

4. Telangiectasia: Spider-like dilations of small vessels

5. Spontaneous bleeds: Mucosal bleeding, such as nose bleeds or gingival bleeds, without inordinate trauma

C. Laboratory evaluation.

1. Tourniquet test: Pressure is increased in small vessels by applying a blood pressure cuff to the patient's arm and inflating it to 80 to 100 mm Hg for 5 minutes. Petechiae form if the vessels are fragile.

2. Bleeding time: Platelets and thrombogenic components of the vessels must interact to form a clot and control bleeding. If either are abnormal, the bleeding time will be prolonged. Elevated bleeding times may also occur after aspirin ingestion. Methods may vary as follows:

   a. Duke bleeding time: The earlobe is the puncture site.

   b. Ivy bleeding time: The forearm is the puncture site and a lancet is used without a template.

   c. Mielke bleeding time: The forearm is the puncture site and a template is used to standardize the incision.

D. Disease states.

1. Aspirin-induced petechiae: Salicylic acid inhibits vasoconstriction leading to pinpoint hemorrhages.

2. Ehlers-Danlos syndrome: Autosomal dominant inheritance of abnormal collagen reduces normal platelet adhesion. The bleeding time may be abnormal.

3. Hereditary hemorrhagic telangiectasia: Au-

tosomal dominant inheritance of a deficiency of elastic fibers results in dilation of capillaries. Bleeding tendencies ensue. The bleeding time is increased, and the tourniquet test is positive.

4. Scurvy: A deficiency of vitamin C results in a decreased level of hyaluronic acid in the basement membrane.

5. Senile purpura: Subcutaneous tissue atrophies as a person ages; thus, vascular support is lacking.

II. The platelets

A. Maturational development in the bone marrow

1. Megakaryoblast: The diameter is 15 to 45 micrometers. The cell has a small amount of deep-blue non-granular cytoplasm which forms cytoplasmic tags but no visible platelets. The finely reticulated nucleus comprises most of the cell and has visible nucleoli.

2. Promegakaryocyte: The diameter is 18 to 65 micrometers. Endomitosis (nuclear division without cellular division) increases the size of the cell, as well as the number of nuclei present in the cell. Nucleoli are visible. The cytoplasm remains blue but contains granules.

3. Megakaryocyte: The diameter is 15 to 55 micrometers. The nucleus is clumped and lobulated with no visible nucleoli. The cytoplasm is abundant and pinkish-purple. Megakaryocytes and metamegakaryocytes may be confused with osteoclasts. The nuclei of osteoclasts may be odd or even in number, whereas the nuclei of megakaryocytic cells are an even number. In addition, the nuclei of osteoclasts are distinct with no connecting filaments as in megakaryocytic cells.

4. Metamegakaryocyte: The diameter is 20 to 50 micrometers. The granulated cytoplasm is lavender with an irregular margin. There may be four or more coarsely clumped nuclei present, but the number will always be even. Bits of granular cytoplasm may be seen at the margin of the cell as platelets form.

5. Platelet: Cytoplasmic fragments of the megakaryocytes are released into the sinusoidal spaces of the bone marrow and eventually into the peripheral blood. Twenty to thirty percent of platelets pool in the spleen and 70 to 80 percent circulate in the blood, where they live for ap-

proximately 10 days. The platelets measure 2 to 4 micrometers in diameter. On a Wright's-stained smear, platelets appear as lavender granulated discs with no nucleus.

B. Platelet structure

1. Peripheral zone: The outermost layer has receptor sites for ADP, collagen, fibrinogen, serotonin, thrombin, von Willebrand's factor, and other thrombogenic agents. An open canalicular system provides a mechanism for secretions and absorptions.

2. Submembrane area: The layer contains the filamentous system which helps maintain the shape of the platelet and separates the organelles from the peripheral zone.

3. Sol-gel zone: The layer contains a system of microtubules and microfilaments which maintain the discoid shape of the platelet until it is stimulated. During platelet shape change, the cytoskeleton contracts.

4. Organelle zone: Dense granules, alpha granules, and other organelles contain substances vital to platelet metabolism, hemostasis, and vessel repair.

C. Platelet kinetics

1. Adhesion: Exposed collagen and subendothelial cells initiate the first step of platelet plug formation. The platelets adhere to surfaces other than platelets. During this step, the platelets change shape from discs to spiny spheres. von Willebrand's factor is required for adhesion.

2. Granule release: The contents of the dense bodies and alpha granules are released. These components facilitate and regulate clot formation.

3. Aggregation: In response to chemical changes in the platelets and to granule release, platelets cohere to other platelets. Aggregating agents include ADP, arachidonic acid, collagen, epinephrine, ristocetin, thrombin, and thromboxane.

4. Stabilization of the clot: Coagulation factors interact with platelet phospholipids to stabilize the clot.

5. Regulators: Arachidonic acid may either be transformed into thromboxane by platelets or into prostacyclin by endothelial cells. Thromboxane is an aggregating agent and a vasoconstrictor. Prostacyclin is an anti-aggregating agent and a vasodilator.

D. Laboratory evaluation

1. Aggregation studies: When an aggregating agent is added to platelet-rich plasma

(PRP), the platelets undergo shape change and aggregation. The reaction allows more light to be transmitted through the suspension. Various aggregating agents cause different aggregation patterns.

2. Antiplatelet antibodies: Immune thrombocytopenias are the result of antibodies against platelet antigens.
3. Bleeding time: See laboratory evaluation of vascular disorders. (See Section IC2.)
4. Clot retraction: If platelet numbers are adequate and platelet function is normal, a clot incubated at 37°C will pull away from the surface of the test tube. At best, the clot retraction test is crude and insensitive.
5. Peripheral blood smear: Eight to 23 platelets per oil immersion field of a wedge-prepared smear should be seen assuming the RBC count is normal. The platelets should be 2 to 4 micrometers in diameter, round, and contain dust-like granules.

6. Platelet counts: Falsely elevated results may occur when RBC inclusions and fragments are present. Falsely decreased results may occur in the presence of platelet clumping and satellitism.
   a. Manual methods: Whole blood is diluted (1:100 or 1:200) with Rees-Ecker solution or 1% ammonium oxalate solution and placed on a hemacytometer. Calculations are performed in accordance with the dilution used, area counted, and depth of the hemacytometer.
   b. Automated methods.
      (1) Electrical impedance: Platelets resist an electrical current between two electrodes. Analog impulses are converted to digital readings.
      (2) Optical: Platelets scatter a light beam and are detected as unique cellular components.
7. Platelet histogram (normal).

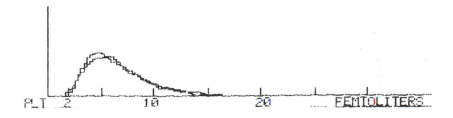

8. Platelet factor 3 availability: Platelets provide a surface for activation of coagulation factors. If platelet factor 3 is unavailable, a clotting time with the patient's PRP remains prolonged.
9. Platelet retention: When whole blood is exposed to glass beads in a column, normal platelets in contact with normal von Willebrand's factor will adhere to the beads. As the blood flows from the column, the platelet count is usually reduced by about 75 percent.

E. Platelet disorders
1. Thrombocytopenia: Clinical manifestations do not usually appear until the platelet count drops below 50×10^9/L. The most severe manifestation is bleeding into the central nervous system.
   a. Decreased production of platelets
      (1) Cause: Such disorders as acute leukemias, marrow aplasia, megaloblastic anemias, and May-Hegglin anomaly reduce platelet numbers.

   (2) Laboratory evaluation.
      (a) Platelet count: Decreased.
      (b) Bone marrow aspiration and biopsy: Megakaryocytes are decreased in aplasia but increased in preleukemic states and megaloblastic anemias.
   b. Increased destruction of platelets
      (1) Immune thrombocytopenic purpura
         (a) Cause: Platelet auto-antibodies may occur following viral infections or may be of unknown origin. Attachment of the antibodies to platelets causes the spleen to destroy the platelets.
         (b) Treatment: Steroids and splenectomy. Platelet transfusions will be ineffective because of antibody attachment to transfused platelets.
         (c) Laboratory evaluation.

(i) Platelet count: Decreased.

(ii) Bleeding time: Increased.

(iii) Tourniquet test: Positive.

(iv) Clot retraction: Poor.

(v) Bone marrow aspiration and biopsy: Increased megakaryocytes without evidence of platelet production will be seen.

(2) Secondary immune thrombocytopenia

(a) Cause: A previously diagnosed autoimmune disorder or drug ingestion may cause antibodies to be formed and attach to platelets. The platelets are then removed by the spleen.

(b) Treatment: Control the underlying disorder, steroids, and plasmapheresis.

(c) Laboratory evaluation.

(i) Platelet count: Decreased.

(ii) Bleeding time: Increased.

(iii) Bone marrow aspiration and biopsy: Megakaryocytes are normal to increased in numbers.

(3) Heparin-associated thrombocytopenia

(a) Cause: The exact mechanism of destruction is unclear, but thrombocytopenia occurs between 1 to 2 weeks after the initiation of heparin therapy.

(b) Treatment: Change sources of heparin or remove the drug.

(c) Laboratory evaluation.

(i) Platelet count: Decreased

(ii) Platelet-associated immunoglobulin: Increased

(4) Thrombotic thrombocytopenic purpura

(a) Cause: Possibly a decreased production of prostacyclin allows intravascular platelet aggregation.

(b) Treatment: Antiplatelet drugs and steroids.

(c) Laboratory evaluation.

(i) Platelet count: Decreased

(ii) RBC count: Decreased

(iii) Peripheral blood smear: Fragmented RBCs

(iv) Bilirubin: Increased

(v) Haptoglobin: Decreased

(vi) Urine hemosiderin: Positive

(vii) Urine hemoglobin: Positive

(5) Disseminated intravascular coagulation

(a) Cause: Introduction of thromboplastin-like substances into the peripheral blood initiates clot formation. Platelets are utilized by the clots.

(b) Treatment: Eliminate the underlying disorder and administer heparin if needed.

(c) Laboratory evaluation.

(i) Platelet count: Decreased

(ii) Fibrinogen: Decreased

(iii) D-Dimer: Positive

(iv) Bleeding time: Increased

(v) Prothrombin time: Increased

(vi) Activated partial thromboplastin time: Increased

c. Abnormal distribution

(1) Cause: An increased number of platelets will pool in an enlarged spleen.

(2) Laboratory evaluation: Platelet count is decreased.

2. Reactive thrombocytosis

a. Cause: Acute blood loss, vigorous exercise, splenectomy, and increased hematopoiesis may cause a transient increase in platelets.

b. Laboratory evaluation.

(1) Platelet count: Increased above 415×10^9/L but usually less than 1000×10^9/L.

(2) Bleeding time: Normal.

(3) Platelet aggregation: Normal.

(4) Bone marrow aspiration and biopsy: Increased number of megakaryocytes.

3. Chronic myeloproliferative disorders

a. Cause: Toxic exposure produces chronic myeloproliferative changes (essential thrombocytopenia, polycythemia vera, chronic myelocytic leukemia, or myeloid metaplasia).

b. Laboratory evaluation.
  (1) Platelet count: Usually exceeds $1000 \times 10^9/L$.
  (2) Bleeding time: Normal to increased.
  (3) Platelet aggregation: Frequently abnormal.
  (4) Bone marrow aspiration and biopsy: Number and size of megakaryocytes are increased.

F. Thrombocytopathies
  1. Bernard-Soulier syndrome
    a. Cause: Autosomal recessive inheritance results in glycoprotein Ib deficiency which is necessary for normal interaction between platelets and von Willebrand's factor.
    b. Laboratory evaluation.
      (1) Platelet count: Decreased
      (2) Bleeding time: Increased
      (3) Clot retraction: Normal
      (4) Aggregation studies: Abnormal with ristocetin but normal with ADP, epinephrine, and arachidonic acid
      (5) Peripheral blood smear: Large platelets
      (6) Platelet factor 3 availability: Normal
      (7) Platelet retention: Decreased
  2. Glanzmann's thrombasthenia
    a. Cause: Autosomal recessive inheritance results in a deficiency of glycoprotein components necessary for platelet aggregation.
    b. Laboratory evaluation.
      (1) Platelet count: Normal
      (2) Bleeding time: Increased
      (3) Clot retraction: Poor
      (4) Platelet retention: Abnormal
      (5) Aggregation studies: Abnormal with ADP, collagen, epinephrine, and thrombin, but normal with ristocetin

  (6) Platelet factor 3 availability: Decreased
  3. Storage pool deficiencies
    a. Cause: Variable inheritance of one of a group of disorders causes a deficiency of platelet granules or a defect in the granules.
    b. Laboratory evaluation.
      (1) Platelet count: Decreased to normal
      (2) Bleeding time: Increased
      (3) Platelet retention: Abnormal
      (4) Platelet factor 3 availability: Decreased
      (5) Platelet secretion: Abnormal
  4. von Willebrand's disease
    a. Cause: Variable inheritance results in abnormal interaction between von Willebrand's factor and platelets.
    b. Laboratory evaluation.
      (1) Platelet count: Normal
      (2) Bleeding time: Increased
      (3) Clot retraction: Poor
      (4) Activated partial thromboplastin time: Normal to increased
      (5) Platelet adhesion: Abnormal
      (6) Aggregation studies: Abnormal with ristocetin
  3. Drug-induced abnormalities
    a. Cause: Drugs, such as aspirin, ethanol, certain antibiotics, and many others, inhibit normal platelet function.
    b. Laboratory evaluation.
      (1) Bleeding time: Increased following aspirin ingestion
      (2) Aggregation studies: Abnormal

REFERENCES

Harmening: 37–38, 415–425, 440–461, 584–592
Lotspeich-Steininger: 565–578, 653–694
McKenzie: 363–380, 417–437
Turgeon: 266–277, 387–390

Chapter 14

Coagulation Mechanisms and Laboratory Evaluation

I. Factor nomenclature: Each factor can be classified as a substrate (the substance on which an enzyme acts), zymogen (enzyme precursor), cofactor (the component that aids in conversion of a zymogen to the active enzyme), or calcium. Once the zymogens are converted to enzymes, they are either serine proteases, which have serine as the active site and cleave peptide bonds, or transaminases, which create covalent bonds. Most factors are produced by the liver and circulate in the peripheral blood in the inactive precursor state. The activated state is designated by the appropriate Roman numeral followed by an "a."

A. Factor I: Fibrinogen is the substrate of the coagulation mechanism. It is composed of three different dimers of polypeptide chains linked by disulfide bridges. Upon cleavage by thrombin, fibrinogen molecules are converted to fibrin monomers which polymerize to form the clot.

B. Factor II: Prothrombin is a serine protease precursor. When activated, it is converted to thrombin which splits fibrinogen, stimulates platelet aggregation, and activates co-factors and protein C.

C. Factor III: Thromboplastin/tissue factor is a cofactor found in tissue. Exceptionally high concentrations are found in the brain and lungs. Factor III activates factor VII when blood is exposed to tissue fluids.

D. Factor IV: Ionized calcium is required at several steps in the coagulation pathway.

E. Factor V: Proaccelerin is the precursor to a cofactor that speeds the transformation of prothrombin to thrombin.

F. Factor VI: Non-existent.

G. Factor VII: Proconvertin is a serine protease precursor which is activated by tissue thromboplastin. After activation, factor VII activates factor X.

H. Factor VIII: Antihemophilic factor A is a cofactor with several functional units.
   1. VIII/vWf is the total factor VIII molecule consisting of a low-molecular-weight unit (VIII) and a high-molecular-weight unit (vWf).
   2. VIII:C is the active portion of the molecule and can be measured by clotting assays.
   3. VIII:Ag is the antigenic portion of the molecule capable of stimulating antibody production and measured by immunoassay.
   4. vWf:Ag is a subunit of VIII/vWf capable of stimulating antibody production and can be measured by immunologic techniques. It is the portion that binds to endothelium and supports normal platelet adhesion and function.

I. Factor IX: Plasma thromboplastin component or antihemophilic factor B, also known as Christmas factor, is a serine protease in the intrinsic coagulation pathway.

J. Factor X: Stuart-Prower factor is a serine protease that converts prothrombin to thrombin.

K. Factor XI: Plasma thromboplastin antecedent is a serine protease that is at the beginning of the intrinsic coagulation pathway.

L. Factor XII: Hageman factor is a serine protease. It can be activated by contact with foreign substances such as collagen.

M. Factor XIII: Fibrin stabilizing factor is a transaminase that stabilizes polymerized fibrin monomers in the initial clot.

N. Prekallikrein: Fletcher factor is converted to kallikrein, a serine protease that connects the coagulation pathways to fibrinolysis and kininogen activation with the help of factor XIIa.

O. High-molecular-weight kininogen: Fitzgerald factor is a cofactor involved in contact activation of the intrinsic coagulation pathway.

II. Coagulation families

A. Fibrinogen family

1. Includes factors I, V, VIII, and XIII.

2. Are consumed during clotting. Therefore, they are present in plasma but not in serum.

3. Decreased in stored plasma due to the lability of factors V and VIII.

4. Do not require vitamin K for synthesis.

5. Are not adsorbed by barium sulfate or aluminum hydroxide; thus, they are present in adsorbed plasma.

6. Are activated by thrombin.

7. Are degraded by plasmin.

B. Prothrombin family

1. Includes factors II, VII, IX, and X.

2. Are not consumed during clotting, with the exception of factor II. Therefore, factors VII, IX, and X are present in plasma and serum.

3. Are stable in stored plasma.

4. Require vitamin K for synthesis of functional factors.

5. Are adsorbed by barium sulfate or aluminum hydroxide; thus, they are not present in adsorbed plasma.

6. Are not activated by thrombin.

7. Are not degraded by plasmin.

C. Contact family

1. Includes factors XI, XII, prekallikrein, and high-molecular-weight kininogen.

2. Are partially consumed during clotting. Therefore, they are present in plasma and serum.

3. Are fairly stable in stored plasma.

4. Do not require vitamin K for synthesis.

5. Are not adsorbed by barium sulfate or aluminum hydroxide; thus, they are present in adsorbed plasma.

6. Are not activated by thrombin.

7. Are not degraded by plasmin.

III. Coagulation mechanisms

A. Intrinsic pathway: Contact with subendothelial tissue initiates the activation of factor XII, factor XI, prekallikrein, and high-molecular-weight kininogen. Factor XIIa not only begins the intrinsic pathway but also interfaces with the fibrinolytic, kinin, and complement systems. Factor XIa converts factor IX into the activated state. With the help of factor VIIIa, the first step in the common pathway is stimulated.

B. Extrinsic pathway: As tissue factor III is released into the blood, it activates factor VII. Factor VIIa stimulates the first step in the common pathway.

C. Common pathway: Factor X may be activated by either the intrinsic or extrinsic pathways. Factor Xa, with the help of factor Va, converts prothrombin to thrombin. In turn, thrombin converts fibrinogen to fibrin monomers which polymerize to form an unstable clot. The clot is stabilized by forming disulfide bonds under the direction of factor XIIIa.

D. Conversion of cofactors and transaminase: The activated state of factors V, VIII, and XIII is initiated by thrombin.

IV. Anticoagulants

A. Natural

1. Antithrombin III (AT III) inhibits thrombin and factors IXa, Xa, XIa, and XIIa. The majority of natural anticoagulant action is controlled by AT III.

2. Naturally occurring heparin and heparan sulfate prevent intravascular clot formation.

3. Proteins C (serine protease) and S (cofactor) work in concert to slow clot formation by inhibiting coagulation cofactors and inactivating inhibitors of plasminogen activators.

4. C1 inactivator inhibits contact factors by inhibiting C1 esterase in the complement pathway.

5. Alpha-2-macroglobulin inhibits the coagulation system as well as the fibrinolytic system.

6. Alpha-1–antitrypsin inhibits factor XIa and thrombin.

B. Acquired

1. Disease states, such as lupus erythematosus, produce inhibitors that hinder the binding of coagulation factors to platelet phospholipids.

2. Drug therapy.

a. Coumarin/warfarin derivatives interfere with the synthesis of the prothrombin family by competing for vitamin K. As these factors decrease, the coagulation mechanism is slowed. Therapy is usually administered orally and may be continued for prolonged periods of time. Coumarin therapy is monitored by the prothrombin time with maximum effect seen 2 to 3 days after initiation of therapy. Likewise, several days may be required for the prothrombin time to return to normal following cessation of therapy.

   b. Heparin enhances the action of AT III; thus, it acts immediately. Heparin's short half-life and administration by intravenous or subcutaneous routes deter long-term usage. Heparin therapy is usually monitored by the activated partial thromboplastin time.

V. Laboratory evaluation of the coagulation mechanism

  A. Caution: Most coagulation tests use platelet-poor plasma from blood anticoagulated at a 9 : 1 ratio with sodium citrate. Volume adjustments must be made with specimens collected from patients with extremely high (>60 percent, 0.60 liters per liter) or extremely low (<20 percent, 0.20 liters per liter) hematocrits. The amount of anticoagulant may be adjusted using the following formula:

$$(0.00185) \ (V) \ (100 - \text{patient's hematocrit in \%}) = C$$

where V = volume of patient's blood in milliliters and C = volume of anticoagulant in milliliters.

  B. Prothrombin time (PT) tests the extrinsic pathway from factor VII to the unstable fibrin clot. The reagent (tissue thromboplastin plus calcium ions) is added to an aliquot of patient plasma. The amount of time for the clot to form is measured electrically or photometrically. Patients receiving coumarin should have a PT between 1.5 to 2 times normal. Normal ranges vary with instrumentation used. Reporting may be as follows:

    1. Patient time in seconds compared to a reference range.

    2. Patient time in seconds compared to a control time.

    3. Patient's percent of normal activity.

    4. PT ratio calculated as follows: Patient time ÷ reference time mean

    5. International normalized ratio (INR): PT ratio[ISI]. The ISI is the international sensitivity index supplied by the manufacturers of thromboplastin reagents.

  C. Activated partial thromboplastin time (APTT) tests the intrinsic pathway from factor XII to the unstable fibrin clot. The reagents (phospholipid and calcium chloride) are added to an aliquot of patient plasma. The reagent has an activator, such as ellagic acid, kaolin, silica, charcoal, or celite, to enhance reproducibility. The amount of time for the clot to form is measured electrically or photometrically. Results are reported in seconds. Patients receiving heparin should have an APTT between 1.5 to 2 times normal.

  D. Common PT/APTT interpretations in the presence of hemostatic abnormalities:

    1. If PT and APTT are normal, the abnormality is probably due to platelet deficiency, vascular defect, or factor XIII deficiency.

    2. If PT is prolonged and APTT is normal, the abnormality is probably due to factor VII deficiency.

    3. If PT is normal and APTT is prolonged, the abnormality is probably due to a deficiency of prekallikrein, high-molecular-weight kininogen, or factors VIII, IX, XI, or XII.

    4. If PT and APTT are prolonged, the abnormality is probably due to a deficiency of factors I, II, V, X, or multiple factor deficiencies. Heparin contamination or a clot in the specimen will also prolong the PT and APTT.

  E. Lee-White whole blood clotting time (LWCT) tests the intrinsic pathway. It is sensitive only to extreme factor deficiencies and exhibits poor reproducibility. Heparin therapy will alter results.

  F. Activated whole blood clotting time tests the intrinsic pathway. Diatomite is added to collection tubes to speed activation of the contact factors. It is more sensitive to factor deficiencies and heparin therapy than the LWCT.

  G. Thrombin time tests the conversion of fibrinogen to fibrin. The reagent (thrombin) is added to an aliquot of patient plasma. The amount of time for the clot to form is measured electrically or photometrically. Heparin and circulating fibrin degradation products will interfere with results.

  H. Fibrinogen assay quantitates the amount of factor I present in plasma. After adding the reagent (thrombin), the clotting time is measured electrically or photometrically and then compared to a previously drawn calibration curve. Results are reported in grams per liter.

  I. Urea (5 M) solubility test checks for the presence of factor XIII. When placed in 5 M urea, a normal plasma clot should not dissolve within 24 hours.

J. Platelet neutralization procedure tests for the presence of a lupus anticoagulant. When platelet extract is added to patient plasma, the APTT should correct if the patient has a lupus anticoagulant.

K. Stypven time (Russell's viper venom time) uses Russell's viper venom as a reagent. The venom contains thromboplastin-like substances which activate factor X without the aid of factor VII. If factor VII is deficient, Russell's viper venom will produce a normal time, but if factor X or any other factor in the common pathway is deficient, the Stypven time will be prolonged.

L. Aspirin tolerance test consists of performing bleeding times before and after aspirin ingestion. Normally, the bleeding time will be slightly prolonged following aspirin inges-tion, but in an individual with von Wille-brand's disease, the bleeding time will be markedly prolonged following aspirin in-take.

M. Substitution studies test for factor deficien-cies. Patient plasma is mixed with either normal plasma, aged serum, or adsorbed plasma prior to testing. If the mixture of normal plasma and patient plasma produce normal PT and APTT, then inhibitors are not present and the abnormal results are caused by a factor deficiency. If factor VII, IX, X, XI, or XII is deficient, aged serum will correct the PT or APTT. If factor I, V, VIII, XI, or XII is deficient, adsorbed plasma will correct the PT or APTT.

N. Factor assay quantitates the factor that is deficient.

REFERENCES

Harmening: 350, 425–439, 498–502, 508–512, 592–609
Lotspeich-Steininger: 568–570, 579–590, 592–595, 599–620, 634, 647–650, 704
McKenzie: 381–402, 406–413, 467–471
Turgeon: 277–286, 383–397

Chapter 15

Coagulation Disorders

I. Hereditary disorders: Usually single factor deficiency

A. Autosomal recessive inheritance: The number of affected males and females in a family will be about equal.

 1. Factor I deficiency

 a. Clinical manifestations: Severe hemorrhaging, hemarthrosis, ecchymoses, epistaxis, and hematomas. Frequently diagnosed at birth due to umbilical stump hemorrhaging.

 b. Laboratory evaluation.

 (1) PT: Increased

 (2) APTT: Increased

 (3) Substitution studies: Corrected with normal plasma and adsorbed plasma but not aged serum

 (4) Thrombin time: Increased

 (5) Fibrinogen assay: Decreased

 (6) Bleeding time: Variable

 c. Treatment: Fresh frozen plasma, cryoprecipitate, or fibrinogen concentrate.

 2. Factor II deficiency

 a. Clinical manifestations: Mild hemorrhaging, ecchymoses, and mucosal bleeding

 b. Laboratory evaluation

 (1) PT: Increased

 (2) APTT: Increased

 (3) Substitution studies: Corrected with normal plasma but not adsorbed plasma or aged serum

 (4) Thrombin time: Normal

 (5) Fibrinogen assay: Normal

 (6) Factor II assay: Decreased

 c. Treatment: Fresh frozen plasma or prothrombin complex concentrates

 3. Factor V deficiency

 a. Clinical manifestations: Mild to moderate bleeding with bruising and epistaxis

 b. Laboratory evaluation

 (1) PT: Increased

 (2) APTT: Increased

 (3) Substitution studies: Corrected with normal plasma and aged serum but not adsorbed plasma

 (4) Thrombin time: Normal

 (5) Fibrinogen assay: Normal

 (6) Stypven time: Increased

 (7) Factor V assay: Decreased

 c. Treatment: Fresh frozen plasma

 4. Factor VII deficiency

 a. Clinical manifestations: Mild to moderate bleeding

 b. Laboratory evaluation

 (1) PT: Increased

 (2) APTT: Normal

 (3) Substitution studies: Corrected with normal plasma and aged serum but not adsorbed plasma

 (4) Stypven time: Normal

 (5) Factor VII assay: Decreased

 c. Treatment: Fresh frozen plasma or prothrombin complex concentrates

 5. Factor X deficiency

 a. Clinical manifestations: Mild to severe bleeding

 b. Laboratory evaluation

 (1) PT: Increased

 (2) APTT: Increased

 (3) Substitution studies: Corrected with normal plasma and aged serum but not adsorbed plasma

 (4) Thrombin time: Normal

 (5) Fibrinogen assay: Normal

 (6) Stypven time: Increased

 (7) Factor X assay: Decreased

 c. Treatment: Fresh frozen plasma or prothrombin complex concentrates

 6. Factor XI deficiency

 a. Clinical manifestations: Mild bleeding after trauma. (Predominately found in the Jewish population.)

 b. Laboratory evaluation.

 (1) PT: Normal

(2) APTT: Increased

(3) Substitution studies: Corrected with normal plasma, aged serum, and adsorbed plasma

(4) Factor XI assay: Decreased

c. Treatment: Fresh frozen plasma.

7. Factor XII deficiency

a. Clinical manifestations: Asymptomatic, thrombosis, or pulmonary emboli.

b. Laboratory evaluation.

(1) PT: Normal

(2) APTT: Increased

(3) Substitution studies: Corrected with normal plasma, aged serum, and adsorbed plasma

(4) Factor XII assay: Decreased

c. Treatment: No therapy is usually required.

8. Factor XIII deficiency

a. Clinical manifestations: Umbilical cord bleeding, delayed healing, and keloid formation

b. Laboratory evaluation

(1) PT: Normal

(2) APTT: Normal

(3) Substitution studies: Corrected with normal plasma and adsorbed plasma but not aged serum

(4) Urea solubility test: Abnormal

(5) Factor XIII assay: Decreased

c. Treatment: Fresh frozen plasma

9. Prekallikrein deficiency

a. Clinical manifestations: Asymptomatic or thrombosis

b. Laboratory evaluation

(1) PT: Normal

(2) APTT: Increased

(3) Substitution studies: Corrected with normal plasma, aged serum, and adsorbed plasma

(4) APTT with extended incubation time: Corrected

(5) Prekallikrein assay: Decreased

c. Treatment: No therapy

10. High-molecular-weight kininogen deficiency

a. Clinical manifestations: Asymptomatic

b. Laboratory evaluation

(1) PT: Normal

(2) APTT: Increased

(3) Substitution studies: Corrected with normal plasma, aged serum, and adsorbed plasma

(4) APTT with extended incubation time: Increased

(5) High-molecular-weight kininogen assay: Decreased

c. Treatment: No therapy

B. Sex-linked recessive inheritance: More males than females in a family are affected.

1. Factor VIII deficiency

a. Clinical manifestations: Mild bleeding and easy bruising to severe hemorrhage, intracranial bleeding, and crippling hemarthrosis

b. Laboratory evaluation

(1) PT: Normal

(2) APTT: Increased

(3) Substitution studies: Corrected with normal plasma, and adsorbed plasma but not aged serum

(4) Bleeding time: Normal

(5) Platelet count: Normal

(6) Platelet aggregation studies: Normal

(7) Factor VIII:C assay: Decreased

(8) Factor VIII:Ag assay: Decreased

(9) vWf:Ag assay: Normal

(10) Factor IX assay: Normal

c. Treatment: Cryoprecipitate, fresh frozen plasma, factor VIII concentrate, or 1-desamino-8-D-arginine vasopressin (DDAVP)

2. Factor IX deficiency

a. Clinical manifestations: Similar to factor VIII deficiency. (See IB1a).

b. Laboratory evaluation

(1) PT: Normal

(2) APTT: Increased

(3) Substitution studies: Corrected with normal plasma and aged serum but not adsorbed plasma

(4) Bleeding time: Normal

(5) Platelet count: Normal

(6) Platelet aggregation studies: Normal

(7) Factor VIII:C assay: Normal

(8) Factor IX assay: Decreased

c. Treatment: Fresh frozen plasma or prothrombin complex concentrates

C. Autosomal dominant inheritance: An equal number of males and females in a family are affected.

1. von Willebrand's disease: May also have autosomal recessive inheritance or be acquired. Several types have been classified according to inheritance patterns and test results.

a. Clinical manifestations: Mild to severe hemorrhaging

b. Laboratory evaluation

(1) PT: Normal

(2) APTT: Normal to increased

(3) Bleeding time: Increased

(4) Aspirin tolerance test: Markedly increased

(5) Platelet count: Normal

(6) Platelet aggregation studies: Abnormal with ristocetin

(7) Factor VIII:C: Normal to decreased

(8) vWf:Ag: Decreased

c. Treatment: Cryoprecipitate or DDAVP

2. Dysfibrinogenemia

a. Clinical manifestations: Asymptomatic to mild bleeding

b. Laboratory evaluation

(1) PT: Variable

(2) APTT: Variable

(3) Thrombin time: Increased

(4) Substitution studies: Corrected with normal plasma and adsorbed plasma but not aged serum

(5) Thrombin time: Increased

(6) Fibrinogen clotting assay: Decreased

(7) Fibrinogen immunologic assay: Normal

c. Treatment: Supportive

3. Antithrombin III (AT III) deficiency

a. Clinical manifestations: Venous thrombosis and pulmonary emboli

b. Laboratory evaluation

(1) PT: Normal

(2) APTT: Normal

(3) AT III assay: Decreased

c. Treatment: Fresh frozen plasma, coumarin, heparin, or AT III concentrates

4. Protein C deficiency

a. Clinical manifestations: Venous thrombosis and pulmonary emboli

b. Laboratory evaluation

(1) PT: Normal

(2) APTT: Normal

(3) Protein C assay: Decreased

c. Treatment: Coumarin, heparin, or factor IX concentrates

5. Protein S deficiency

a. Clinical manifestations: Venous thrombosis

b. Laboratory evaluation

(1) PT: Normal

(2) APTT: Normal

(3) Protein S assay: Decreased

c. Treatment: Coumarin

II. Acquired disorders: Usually multiple factor deficiencies

A. Liver disease

1. Cause: Since most coagulation factors are synthesized in the liver, liver disease causes decreased synthesis of these factors.

2. Clinical manifestations: Hemorrhage, purpura, and petechiae.

3. Laboratory evaluation.

a. Liver enzymes: Increased

b. Bilirubin: Increased

c. PT: Increased

d. APTT: Variable

e. Peripheral blood smear: Codocytes (target cells)

4. Treatment: Supportive.

B. Hemorrhagic disease of the newborn

1. Cause: The infant has an immature liver, limited vitamin K storage, and inadequate vitamin K–producing intestinal flora; thus, functional factors in the prothrombin family cannot be synthesized.

2. Clinical manifestations: Umbilical stump bleeding, cephalhematoma, and bleeding after circumcision.

3. Laboratory evaluation.

a. PT: Increased

b. APTT: Normal to increased

c. Bleeding time: Normal

d. Platelet count: Normal

4. Treatment: Vitamin K administration.

C. Sterile gut syndrome

1. Cause: Antibiotics may eliminate normal intestinal flora that produce vitamin K; thus, functional factors in the prothrombin family cannot be synthesized.

2. Clinical manifestations: Oozing from venipuncture sites and mucosal bleeding.

3. Laboratory evaluation.

a. PT: Increased

b. APTT: Increased

4. Treatment: Vitamin K administration.

D. Malabsorption of fats

1. Cause: Vitamin K is a fat-soluble vitamin; thus, if fats are not available due to biliary obstruction, prolonged diarrhea, or intestinal disease, functional factors in the prothrombin family cannot be synthesized.

2. Clinical manifestations: Bleeding.

3. Laboratory evaluation.

a. PT: Increased

b. APTT: Increased

4. Treatment: Vitamin K administration.

E. Disseminated intravascular coagulation (DIC)

1. Cause: DIC is secondary to a disorder that causes thrombus formation throughout the vasculature. Platelets and coagulation factors are depleted by the clotting process

which also activates the fibrinolytic system. This consumption and fibrinolysis leads to hemorrhage.

2. Clinical manifestations: Purpura and bleeding.
3. Laboratory evaluation.
   a. PT: Increased
   b. APTT: Increased
   c. Fibrinogen assay: Decreased
   d. Platelet count: Decreased
   e. Fibrin(ogen) split products: Positive
   f. D-Dimer: Positive
   g. Peripheral blood smear: Fragmented RBCs
4. Treatment: Elimination or control of the primary disorder.

REFERENCES

Harmening: 462–485, 489–497
Lotspeich-Steininger: 584, 626–635, 639–646
McKenzie: 437–467
Turgeon: 286–297

Chapter 16

The Fibrinolytic System

I. Components
  A. Plasminogen: Inert precursor glycoprotein (zymogen) which may be converted to plasmin by fibrinolytic activators.
  B. Plasmin: Serine protease that results when plasminogen is activated. The enzyme degrades factors I, V, VIII, XIIa, XIII, and fibrin. In addition, it activates the complement pathway and the kinin system.
  C. Activators.
    1. Naturally occurring serine proteases
      a. tPA is a serine protease synthesized by the endothelium. It is probably regulated by activated protein C, but the exact mechanism is unknown.
      b. Urokinase is a proteolytic enzyme found in body fluids.
      c. Factor XIIa, kallikrein, high-molecular-weight kininogen, and a proactivator combine to activate the fibrinolytic system.
    2. Acquired therapeutic agents: Often monitored with the thrombin time. Therapeutic range is 1.5 to 5 times the reference range.
      a. tPA is produced by recombinant DNA techniques and used to induce fibrinolysis.
      b. Urokinase is purified from urine and used to activate fibrinolysis.
      c. Streptokinase is isolated from beta-hemolytic streptococci. It functions like the activators of human origin but is more antigenic.
      d. Staphylokinase is isolated from staphylococci. It functions like the activators of human origin but is more antigenic.
  D. Inhibitors.
    1. Naturally occurring.
      a. Alpha-2-antiplasmin irreversibly attaches to free plasmin rendering plasmin non-functional.
      b. Alpha-2-macroglobulin inhibits fibrinolysis when alpha-2-antiplasmin is depleted.
      c. Alpha-1-antitrypsin inhibits fibrinolysis when alpha-2-antiplasmin and alpha-2-macroglobulin are depleted.
    2. Acquired therapeutic agents: Epsilon-aminocaproic acid (EACA) inhibits plasminogen activators and, to a slight degree, plasmin.

II. Fibrinolytic mechanism: Fibrinolysis may be activated intrinsically by the activated contact factors of the coagulation pathway or extrinsically by tissue activators, such as tPA or urokinase. When plasmin is formed, it degrades fibrinogen, fibrin, factor V, factor VIII, and factor XIII. Fibrinogen and fibrin are cleaved to produce a clottable molecule known as fragment X. Fragment X is further degraded to fragments Y and D. Fragment Y is further degraded to fragment E and an additional D fragment. The term fibrin(ogen) split products is used to indicate the by-products of fibrinogen *and* fibrin breakdown. When by-products of only fibrin are indicated, they are known as fibrin split products or D-dimers. Fibrin(ogen) split products (FSPs) may act as circulating anticoagulants until cleared by the liver and other organs. FSPs are also known as fibrin(ogen) degradation products (FDPs).

III. Laboratory testing for fibrinolysis
  A. Whole blood clot lysis: A clot incubated at 37°C for 48 hours should not show significant lysis.
  B. Euglobulin lysis time: Fibrinogen, plasminogen, plasmin, and fibrinolytic activators are precipitated from plasma and then clotted. The clot should remain intact for 2 to 4 hours.
  C. Protamine sulfate test: If present in plasma, fibrin monomers and FSPs can be precipitated by protamine sulfate.
  D. Fibrin(ogen) split products assay: Latex particles are coated with antibodies to FSPs. If a

significant level of the fragments are in the serum, agglutination will occur.

E. D-Dimer assay: Crosslinked D-dimer fragments result when stabilized fibrin clots are degraded by plasmin. Monoclonal antibodies to D-dimers are attached to latex particles causing agglutination if D-dimers are present.

F. Plasminogen assay: Chromogenic or fluorogenic substrates allow functional quantitation of plasminogen.

G. Fibrinopeptides A or B assay: Fibrinogen fragments can be measured by radioimmunoassay.

IV. Disorders

A. Congenital

1. Plasminogen deficiency results in recurrent thrombosis and pulmonary emboli.

2. Activator deficiencies result in recurrent thrombosis.

3. Inhibitor deficiencies result in bleeding episodes.

B. Acquired

1. Primary fibrinolysis: Plasmin activity is increased due to an excess of plasminogen activators. No evidence of previous clots exists. The fibrinogen family is degraded by plasmin.

    a. Cause

    (1) Severe liver disease: Activators are normally cleared from the blood by the liver; therefore, in severe liver disease, activators increase and fibrinolysis is initiated.

    (2) Malignant tumor: Activators increase in the peripheral circulation with fibrinolytic activation resulting.

    b. Clinical manifestations: Bleeding

    c. Laboratory evaluation

    (1) PT: Increased

    (2) APTT: Increased

    (3) Thrombin time: Increased

    (4) Fibrinogen assay: Decreased

    (5) Platelet count: Normal to slightly decreased

    (6) Bleeding time: Normal

    (7) Peripheral blood smear: Normal RBC morphology

    (8) Euglobulin lysis time: Markedly decreased

    (9) FSP assay: Positive

    (10) D-Dimer assay: Negative

    (11) Protamine sulfate: Negative

    d. Treatment: Natural antiplasmins, EACA, or trans-p-aminomethyl-cyclohexanecarboxylic acid (AMCA)

2. Secondary fibrinolysis.

    a. Cause: Excessive fibrin formation from such disorders as disseminated intravascular coagulation activates the fibrinolytic system. The fibrinogen family, prothrombin, and platelets are consumed in the clots. Secondary fibrinolysis is much more common than primary fibrinolysis.

    b. Clinical manifestations: Thrombosis or bleeding

    c. Laboratory evaluation

    (1) PT: Increased

    (2) APTT: Increased

    (3) Thrombin time: Increased

    (4) Fibrinogen assay: Decreased

    (5) Platelet count: Moderately decreased

    (6) Bleeding time: Increased

    (7) Peripheral blood smear: Schizocytes (schistocytes) and spherocytes

    (8) Euglobulin lysis time: Normal to decreased

    (9) FSP assay: Positive

    (10) D-Dimer assay: Positive

    (11) Protamine sulfate: Positive

    d. Treatment: Eliminate the underlying disorder if possible.

REFERENCES

Harmening: 430–435, 486–505, 609–617
Lotspeich-Steininger: 590–592, 595–598, 621–625, 635–638, 642
McKenzie: 402–406, 413–416, 455–458, 466, 471
Turgeon: 289–292, 390–391, 393–395

Section Three
Worksheets

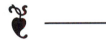

1. A. Blood is pipetted to the 1.0 mark of the RBC pipet, and the number of platelets counted in the center primary square equals 296. Calculate the platelet count.

   B. Is this consistent with normal adult values?

2. A. Blood is pipetted to the 0.5 mark of the RBC pipet, and the number of platelets counted in the center primary square on both sides of the hemacytometer equals 90. Calculate the platelet count.

   B. Is this consistent with normal adult values?

3. The following laboratory data were obtained on a 55-year-old black male with polycythemia vera:

   RBC = $6.59 \times 10^6/\mu L$ or $6.59 \times 10^{12}/L$
   Hb = 21.1 g/dL or 211 g/L
   Hct = 62.4% or 0.624 L/L

   A. Calculate the appropriate amount of blood to be collected for a prothrombin time if 0.5 mL of sodium citrate is in the specimen collection tube.

   B. Calculate the amount of anticoagulant needed if 4.5 mL of blood is to be collected.

4. List at least four common symptoms associated with platelet defects.

5. Identify at least four laboratory tests that are used to evaluate platelet disorders.

6. Interpret the data for the following patients by identifying the most probable platelet disorder.

Laboratory Test	Normal Range	Patient A	Patient B	Patient C
Patient data		54-year-old female with carcinoma of the lung, ecchymoses, and post-surgical oozing from the operative site.	7-year-old male with bleeding following removal of tonsils. Family has a history of bleeding disorders.	5-year-old female with multiple petechiae and purpura. She had the measles 2 weeks ago.
WBC ($\times 10^9$/L)	4.5–11.0	11.0	14.3	8.8
Hemoglobin (g/L)	Male: 135–180 Female: 120–160	89	105	125
Platelet count ($\times 10^9$/L)	140–415	35	165	24
Prothrombin time (s)	10.0–14.0	18.5	12.1	11.7
Activated partial thromboplastin time (s)	22–40	63	41	28
Thrombin time (s)	8–15	30	18	15
Fibrinogen (mg/dL)	155–405	105	257	315
Euglobulin lysis time (min)	No lysis in 120 min	90	Not done	Not done
D-Dimer (μg/mL)	<0.5	>1.0	Not done	<0.5
Bleeding time (min)	2–9	13.0	15.5	18.0
Factor VIII assay (%)	50–150	Not done	45	Not done
Platelet aggregation studies	Normal	Not done	Abnormal with ristocetin	Not done
Miscellaneous tests		Schizocytes (schistocytes) on the blood smear.	No specific findings.	Increased megakaryocytes in the bone marrow.
Interpretation				

7. Define the following:

   A. Thrombocytopathy

   B. Thrombocytosis

C. Thrombocytopenia

8. Match the coagulation factor with the appropriate name. Each name may be used only once.

A. _____ Factor I
B. _____ Factor II
C. _____ Factor III
D. _____ Factor IV
E. _____ Factor V
F. _____ Factor VI
G. _____ Factor VII
H. _____ Factor VII
I. _____ Factor IX
J. _____ Factor X
K. _____ Factor XI
L. _____ Factor XII
M. _____ Factor XIII
N. _____ Prekallikrein
O. _____ High-molecular-weight kininogen

a. Calcium
b. Fibrinogen
c. Prothrombin
d. Tissue thromboplastin
e. Fitzgerald factor
f. Fletcher factor
g. Hageman factor
h. Antihemophilic factor
i. Plasma thromboplastin antecedent
j. Christmas factor
k. Stable factor (proconvertin)
l. Stuart-Prower factor
m. Labile factor (proaccelerin)
n. Fibrin-stabilizing factor
o. No assigned name

9. Identify the most probable factor deficiency based on the following laboratory results. (N = normal; AB = abnormal; C = corrected; NC = not corrected; n/a = not applicable)

Laboratory Test	Patient A	Patient B	Patient C	Patient D	Patient E	Patient F
PT	N	N	AB	AB	AB	AB
APTT	AB	AB	N	AB	AB	AB
Adsorbed plasma PT	n/a	n/a	NC	NC	C	NC
Aged serum PT	n/a	n/a	C	NC	NC	C
Adsorbed plasma APTT	C	NC	n/a	NC	C	NC
Aged serum APTT	NC	C	n/a	NC	NC	C
Interpretation						

10. State the formula for calculation of the international normalized ratio (INR).

11. Calculate the INR for the following patients.

  A. PT = 18.0 s, control = 11.5 s, ISI = 1.3

  B. PT = 15.7 s, control = 11.5 s, ISI = 1.2

12. Match the test on the left with the purpose of the test on the right. Each answer may be used only once.

  A. _____ Bleeding time

  B. _____ Platelet retention

  C. _____ Platelet aggregation

  D. _____ Activated partial thromboplastin time

  E. _____ Prothrombin time

  F. _____ Stypven time

  G. _____ Thrombin time

  H. _____ Platelet neutralization

  I. _____ D-Dimer

  a. Screens abnormalities in the intrinsic coagulation pathway

  b. Identifies a lupus anticoagulant

  c. Evaluates quantitative and qualitative fibrinogen defects

  d. Measures the ability of platelets to inhibit bleeding in vivo

  e. Identifies disease states in which fibrinolysis is occurring

  f. Measures the ability of platelets to adhere to other platelets

  g. Screens abnormalities in the extrinsic coagulation pathway

  h. Measures the ability of platelets to adhere to glass beads

  i. Differentiates between deficiencies of factors VII and X

13. List in order the steps involved in the formation of a hemostatic platelet plug.

14. Each of the following patients has a bleeding problem. Identify the coagulation factors and/or other hemostatic disorders that would be consistent with the results.

Laboratory Test	Normal Range	Patient A	Patient B	Patient C	Patient D
PT (s)	10.0–14.0	32.0	11.5	11.1	18.4
APTT (s)	22–40	31	78	28	52
Interpretation					

15. A 6-year-old male was admitted for a coagulation work-up. He had a history of prolonged bleeding after minor trauma. An older sister had a similar history. Two other siblings and parents were clinically normal. The initial screening tests were as follows:

Laboratory Test	Normal Range	Patient
PT (s)	10.0–14.0	46.8
APTT (s)	22–40	105
Thrombin time (s)	8–15	13.8
Bleeding time (min)	2–9	6.5
Platelet count ($\times 10^9$/L)	140–415	303

A. Identify the coagulation factors that may be deficient.

B. State the probable mode of inheritance such as autosomal dominant.

C. Based on the following mixing studies, identify the most likely coagulation factor deficiency.

Laboratory Test	Patient + Aged Serum	Patient + Adsorbed Plasma
PT (s)	44.4	11.9
APTT (s)	103	31

D. How could this deficiency be confirmed?

16. A 9-month-old male was seen in the emergency department with ecchymoses following a fall from a chair. His maternal grandfather had "bleeding episodes." No other history of bleeding was noted. The initial work-up revealed the following results:

Laboratory Test	Normal Range	Patient
PT (s)	10.0–14.0	11.2
APTT (s)	22–40	90
Bleeding time (min)	2–9	5.0
Platelet count ($\times 10^9$/L)	140–415	263

A. Identify the coagulation factors that may be deficient.

B. Based on the clinical history, which deficiencies identified in part A are unlikely?

C. Based on the following mixing studies, identify the most likely coagulation factor deficiency.

Laboratory Test	Patient + Aged Serum	Patient + Adsorbed Plasma
APTT (in seconds)	35	87

D. Does the history support the mode of inheritance for this deficiency?

17. Match the most likely coagulation problem on the right with the coagulation test on the left. Each answer may be used only once.

A. _____ Abnormal urea solubility test

B. _____ Correction of prolonged APTT when the incubation time is increased or kaolin is added

C. _____ Prolonged thrombin time

D. _____ Inadequate correction of prolonged PT or APTT when patient plasma is mixed with normal plasma

E. _____ Normal platelet aggregation with all reagents except ristocetin

a. Factor I deficiency

b. Factor XIII deficiency

c. von Willebrand's disease

d. Hemophilia A

e. Prekallikrein deficiency

f. Factor inhibitors

18. Name the five molecular components of the fibrinolytic system.

19. Briefly define disseminated intravascular coagulation (DIC).

20. List at least five conditions that may be associated with DIC.

21. Explain the interaction of the coagulation and fibrinolytic systems.

22. Name at least three fibrinolytic inhibitors.

23. Complete the following chart by identifying the typical laboratory findings in decompensated disseminated intravascular coagulation (secondary fibrinolysis) and primary fibrinolysis. Use "↑" for increased, "↓" for decreased, "nl" for normal, "+" for positive, "−" for negative, or other descriptive terms as needed.

Laboratory Test	Disseminated Intravascular Coagulation	Primary Fibrinolysis
Peripheral RBC morphology		
PT		
APTT		
Thrombin time		
Platelet count		
Bleeding time		
Euglobulin lysis time		
Protamine sulfate test		
Fibrin(ogen) split products		
D-Dimer		
Fibrinogen		
Antithrombin III		

Answers to Section Three Worksheets

1. A. Cells counted = 296
   Dilution = 1 : 100; therefore the reciprocal is 100
   Area = 1 × 1 = 1; therefore the reciprocal is 1
   Depth = 1/10; therefore the reciprocal is 10
   Actual cell count = (296)(100)(1)(10)
   $$= 296 \times 10^3/mm^3 \text{ or } 296 \times 10^9/L$$

   B. Yes
   REF: H:525 – 529; L:318 – 322, 672; M:x; T:348 – 349

2. A. Cells counted = 90
   Dilution = 1 : 200; therefore the reciprocal is 200
   Area = 1 × 1 × 2 = 2; therefore the reciprocal is 1/2 or 0.5
   Depth = 1/10; therefore the reciprocal is 10
   Actual cell count = (90)(200)(0.5)(10)
   $$= 90 \times 10^3/mm^3 \text{ or } 90 \times 10^9/L$$

   B. No
   REF: H:525 – 529; L:318 – 322, 672; M:x; T:348 – 349

3. A. 0.5 = (0.00185)(V)(100 − 62.4)
   V = 7.2 mL of blood
   B. C = (0.00185)(4.5)(100 − 62.4) = 0.3 mL of anticoagulant
   REF: H:350; L:x; M:407; T:384

4. Epistaxis, petechiae, purpura, ecchymoses, hematuria, menorrhagia, gastrointestinal bleeding, excessive
   bleeding from cuts, spontaneous gingival bleeding, central nervous system bleeding
   REF: H:441; L:680 – 681; M:418; T:273

5. Bleeding time, platelet count, platelet morphology, platelet aggregation, platelet adhesion, platelet
   secretion, platelet aggregometry
   REF: H:441; L:681, 689 – 690; M:376, 432 – 436; T:276 – 277

6. A. Disseminated intravascular coagulation. REF: H:585 – 612; L:635; M:457; T:291
   B. von Willebrand's disease. REF: H:585 – 612; L:630; M:443; T:287 – 289
   C. Autoimmune or idiopathic thrombocytopenic purpura. REF: H:585 – 612; L:684; M:425; T:274

7. A. Qualitative disorder of platelet function. REF: H:441; L:689; M:x; T:275
   B. Increased platelet count. REF: H:448; L:680; M:430; T:275
   C. Decreased platelet count. REF: H:448; L:680; M:424; T:273

8. A. b
    B. c
    C. d
    D. a
    E. m
    F. o
    G. k
    H. h
    I. j
    J. l
    K. i
    L. g
    M. n
    N. f
    O. e
    REF: H:426; L:582; M:382; T:278

9. A. VIII
    B. IX
    C. VII
    D. II
    E. V
    F. X
    REF: H:432; L:613; M:412; T:392

10. $\text{INR} = \left[\dfrac{\text{patient value (in seconds)}}{\text{reference mean (in seconds)}} \right]^{\text{International Sensitivity Index}}$

    REF: H:510; L:704; M:x; T:x

11. A. $\text{INR} = (18.0 \div 11.5)^{1.3} = 1.8$
    B. $\text{INR} = (15.7 \div 11.5)^{1.2} = 1.5$
    REF: H:510; L:704; M:x; T:x

12. A. d. REF: H:585; L:673; M:376; T:387
    B. h. REF: H:588; L:673; M:x; T:x
    C. f. REF: H:589; L:675; M:378; T:327
    D. a. REF: H:593; L:608; M:409; T:385
    E. g. REF: H:594; L:609; M:408; T:396
    F. i. REF: H:596; L:632; M:395; T:x
    G. c. REF: H:597; L:613; M:411; T:396
    H. b. REF: H:608; L:616; M:x; T:x
    I. e. REF: H:610; L:623; M:x; T:x

13. Endothelium injury, platelet adhesion, platelet aggregation, platelet granule release, fibrin formation and polymerization, clot stabilization
    REF: H:425; L:663–667; M:371; T:273

14. A. Factor VII deficiency. REF: H:481; L:613; M:450; T:392

   B. Deficiency of factor VIII, IX, XI, XII, prekallikrein, high-molecular-weight kininogen, or the presence of inhibitors to these factors. REF: H:481; L:613, 627; M:439; T:283

   C. Factor XIII deficiency, platelet disorders, or vessel fragility. REF: H:482; L:608, 613; M:450; T:275, 283

   D. Deficiency of factor I, II, V, X, multiple factor deficiencies, or the presence of inhibitors to these factors. REF: H:481 – 482; L:613; M:439; T:283

15. A. II, V, and X. REF: H:482; L:613; M:450; T:283, 392

   B. Autosomal recessive. REF: H:475; L:53; M:449 – 454; T:x

   C. V (Note: One third of patients with this deficiency may present with an elevated bleeding time.) REF: H:482; L:613; M:412; T:392

   D. Factor V assay. REF: H:475; L:632; M:452; T:392

16. A. VIII, IX, XI, XII, prekallikrein, and high-molecular-weight kininogen. REF: H:482; L:613, 627; M:439; T:283, 392

   B. Deficiency of factor XII, prekallikrein, or high-molecular-weight kininogen, since patients with one of these deficiencies are asymptomatic or thrombotic. REF: H:465; L:627; M:452 – 454; T:289

   C. IX. REF: H:482; L:613; M:412; T:392

   D. Yes, sex-linked recessive. REF: H:472; L:629; M:446; T:x

17. A. b. REF: H:477; L:633; M:413; T:394

   B. e. REF: H:477; L:627; M:454; T:x

   C. a. REF: H:474; L:613; M:450; T:396

   D. f. REF: H:483; L:615; M:459 – 461; T:292

   E. c. REF: H:470; L:630; M:443; T:289

18. Plasminogen, plasminogen activators, plasmin, plasmin inhibitors, fibrin/fibrinogen
   REF: H:486 – 487; L:590 – 591; M:402; T:282

19. DIC is characterized by consumption of the coagulation factors and platelets to such a degree that the anticoagulant factors no longer outweigh the procoagulant factors, which results in formation of fibrin thrombi throughout the blood vessels. REF: H:489; L:635; M:455; T:291

20. Burns, shock, sepsis, acidosis, pregnancy, heat stroke, liver disease, physical trauma, anoxia or hypoxia, certain snake bites, certain malignancies, certain immunologic conditions
   REF: H:491; L:635; M:456; T:290

21. The contact phase of coagulation requires factors XI and XII, prekallikrein, and high-molecular-weight kininogen. These components interact with each other and activate plasminogen to plasmin. REF: H:488; L:587 – 592; M:405; T:280 – 282

22. Antithrombin III, protein C, protein S, heparin cofactor, alpha-2-macroglobulin, alpha-1-antitrypsin, C1 inactivator
   REF: H:500 – 502; L:592 – 595; M:400; T:284 – 286

23.

Laboratory Test	Disseminated Intravascular Coagulation	Primary Fibrinolysis
Peripheral RBC morphology	RBC fragmentation	nl
PT	↑	↑
APTT	↑	↑
Thrombin time	↑	↑
Platelet count	↓	nl
Bleeding time	↑	nl
Euglobulin lysis time	Variable	↓
Protamine sulfate test	+	−
Fibrin(ogen) split products	↑	↑
D-Dimer	↑	nl
Fibrinogen	↓	↓
Anti-thrombin-III	↓	nl

REF: H:492–495; L:635–636; M:457; T:290–292

Section Three Questions

Select the Best Answer	Answers & References
1. Platelets circulate in the peripheral blood for approximately _____ days.	B
A. 3	H:417
B. 9	L:663
C. 28	M:368
D. 45	T:271
2. Platelets carry:	D
A. Platelet factors only.	H:419
B. Coagulation factor V only.	L:666
C. Coagulation factors V and VIII only.	M:369
D. Coagulation factors V and VIII and platelet factors.	T:x
3. The contractile area of platelets is the _____ zone.	B
A. Peripheral	H:418
B. Sol-gel	L:661
C. Organelle	M:369
D. Ultrastructural	T:271
4. The metabolic area of platelets is the _____ zone.	C
A. Peripheral	H:418
B. Sol-gel	L:660
C. Organelle	M:369
D. Ultrastructural	T:x
5. Platelet adhesion requires the presence of:	A
A. von Willebrand factor.	H:421
B. Fibrinogen.	L:664
C. Calcium.	M:372
D. Thrombin.	T:272

Select the Best Answer	Answers & References

6. Dense granules of platelets release:
    A. Serotonin and calcium.
    B. ADP, calcium, and fibrinogen.
    C. Calcium and fibrinogen.
    D. ADP, calcium, and serotonin.
	D
	H:424
	L:661
	M:370
	T:271

7. Which of the following causes irreversible inactivation of platelets?
    A. Acetaminophen
    B. Heparin
    C. Coumadin
    D. Aspirin
	D
	H:424
	L:650
	M:437
	T:273

8. A normal bleeding time is usually present in:
    A. Vascular disorders.
    B. Quantitative platelet disorders.
    C. Qualitative platelet disorders.
    D. Factor IX deficiency.
	D
	H:436
	L:673
	M:377–378
	T:x

9. Which of the following are platelet adhesion disorders?
    A. von Willebrand's disease and Glanzmann's thrombasthenia
    B. von Willebrand's disease and Bernard-Soulier syndrome
    C. Glanzmann's thrombasthenia and Bernard-Soulier syndrome
    D. Glanzmann's thrombasthenia and Hermansky-Pudlak syndrome
	B
	H:441
	L:689–690
	M:432–435
	T:276

10. Which of the following are platelet aggregation disorders?
    A. Wiskott-Aldrich syndrome and Chédiak-Higashi syndrome
    B. von Willebrand's disease and Bernard-Soulier syndrome
    C. Glanzmann's thrombasthenia and Bernard-Soulier syndrome
    D. Glanzmann's thrombasthenia and congenital afibrinogenemia
	D
	H:441
	L:690
	M:435
	T:276

11. Which of the following describes Bernard-Soulier syndrome?
    A. Prolonged bleeding time and giant platelets
    B. Defective platelet secretion and abnormal clot retraction
    C. Abnormal platelet–vessel wall interaction
    D. Megakaryocytic hyperplasia and splenomegaly
	A
	H:443
	L:690
	M:433–435
	T:273

12. Which of the following describes Glanzmann's thrombasthenia?
    A. Abnormality of glycoproteins IIb and IIIa
    B. Defects in platelet secretion
    C. Abnormal platelet–vessel wall interaction
    D. Abnormality of glycoprotein Ib and platelet adhesion
	A
	H:443
	L:691
	M:435
	T:276

Select the Best Answer	Answers & References

13. Fever, pallor, thrombocytopenia, renal damage, microangiopathic hemolytic anemia, and neurologic deficits are characteristics of:
   A. Decompensated DIC.
   B. Compensated DIC.
   C. Hypercoagulability secondary to liver disease.
   D. Thrombotic thrombocytopenic purpura.
	D
	H:495
	L:682
	M:226
	T:274

14. Most if not all of the coagulation factors are produced in the:
   A. Liver.
   B. Spleen.
   C. Bone-marrow.
   D. Lymph nodes.
	A
	H:432
	L:583
	M:383
	T:277

15. Which of the following are present in adsorbed plasma?
   A. Factors II and IX
   B. Factors II and XI
   C. Factors IX and X
   D. Factors XI and XII
	D
	H:426
	L:613
	M:410
	T:278

16. The prothrombin time screens for abnormalities in which pathway(s)?
   A. Extrinsic
   B. Intrinsic
   C. Extrinsic and intrinsic
   D. Common
	A
	H:428
	L:609
	M:408
	T:283

17. The activated partial thromboplastin time screens for abnormalities in which pathway(s)?
   A. Extrinsic
   B. Intrinsic
   C. Extrinsic and intrinsic
   D. Common
	B
	H:428
	L:608
	M:409
	T:283

18. Which of the following are adsorbed by barium sulfate?
   A. Contact factors
   B. Prothrombin factors
   C. Fibrinogen factors
   D. Fibrinogen factors and the prothrombin factors
	B
	H:426
	L:583
	M:386
	T:278

19. Which of the following coagulation factors are labile at room temperature?
   A. I and II
   B. II and III
   C. III and V
   D. V and VIII
	D
	H:432–433
	L:585
	M:384
	T:278

Select the Best Answer	Answers & References

20. Which of the following coagulation factors is *not* vitamin K-dependent?
    A. VII
    B. VIII
    C. IX
    D. X
	B
	H:432
	L:583
	M:386
	T:287

21. Which of the following is required in the extrinsic, intrinsic, and common pathways?
    A. V
    B. VII
    C. VIII
    D. Calcium
	D
	H:427
	L:581
	M:387
	T:280–281

22. The factor deficiency that causes an abnormal PT but does not affect the APTT is factor:
    A. VII.
    B. VIII.
    C. IX.
    D. X.
	A
	H:482
	L:613
	M:439
	T:392

23. An abnormal APTT and normal PT would be consistent with all of the following factor deficiencies *except* factor:
    A. VIII.
    B. IX.
    C. X.
    D. XI.
	C
	H:482
	L:613
	M:439
	T:392

24. The most sensitive index of heparin therapy and DIC is the:
    A. PT.
    B. APTT.
    C. Bleeding time.
    D. Thrombin time.
	D
	H:481
	L:614
	M:411
	T:283

25. Antithrombin III is enhanced by:
    A. Serine protease.
    B. Heparin.
    C. Plasmin.
    D. Plasminogen.
	B
	H:500
	L:593
	M:401
	T:284

26. Coumadin:
    A. Alters the synthesis of vitamin K–dependent clotting factors.
    B. Reduces the circulating levels of factors II, V, and X.
    C. Reduces the circulating level of factor I.
    D. Cleaves carboxyreductase to generate glutamic acid.
	A
	H:508
	L:649
	M:470
	T:x

Select the Best Answer	Answers & References

27. The most common laboratory test to monitor oral anticoagulant therapy is the:
    A. PT.
    B. APTT.
    C. Thrombin time.
    D. Bleeding time.
	A
	H:509
	L:650
	M:470
	T:283

28. Heparin:
    A. Cleaves phospholipids to generate coagulase.
    B. Binds with heparin cofactor to produce heparin cofactor II.
    C. Cleaves oligosaccharides into D-glucosamine.
    D. Binds with antithrombin III to inhibit thrombin.
	D
	H:510
	L:648
	M:468
	T:284

29. The most common laboratory test to monitor heparin therapy is the:
    A. PT.
    B. APTT.
    C. Thrombin time.
    D. Bleeding time.
	B
	H:512
	L:649
	M:469
	T:386

30. Which of the following are decreased in von Willebrand's disease?
    A. VIII and vWF
    B. VIII, IX, XI, vWF, and ristocetin cofactor activity
    C. VIII, vWF, vWF:Ag, and ristocetin cofactor activity
    D. VIII, IX, XI, vWF:Ag, and ristocetin cofactor activity
	C
	H:441
	L:630
	M:443
	T:290

31. A deficiency of which factor is associated with an asymptomatic or thrombotic presentation?
    A. I
    B. II
    C. XII
    D. XIII
	C
	H:465
	L:627
	M:450
	T:289

32. Which of the following is (are) a sex-linked disorder(s)?
    A. Hemophilia A
    B. von Willebrand's disease
    C. Hemophilia A and von Willebrand's disease
    D. von Willebrand's disease and afibrinogenemia
	A
	H:466
	L:628, 630
	M:439, 446
	T:287

33. Which of the following are usually abnormal in hemophilia A?
    A. PT and APTT
    B. APTT and factor VIII level
    C. Factor VIII level and vWF:Ag
    D. APTT, factor VIII level, and vWF:Ag
	B
	H:470
	L:628
	M:443
	T:290

Select the Best Answer	Answers & References

34. Which of the following are usually abnormal in von Willebrand's disease?
 	
    A. PT and APTT
    B. PT, APTT, and factor VIII level
    C. PT and vWF:Ag
    D. APTT, factor VIII level, and vWF:Ag
	D
	
	H:470
	L:630
	M:443
	T:290

	Bleeding Time	Reptilase Time	Thrombin Time
a	Abnormal	Abnormal	Abnormal
b	Normal	Abnormal	Abnormal
c	Abnormal	Normal	Abnormal
d	Abnormal	Abnormal	Normal

Select the Best Answer	Answers & References

35. Which of the above results correspond to afibrinogenemia?
 	
    A. a
    B. b
    C. c
    D. d
	A
	
	H:474
	L:614–615, 673
	M:450
	T:x

36. Hereditary thrombotic disorders include:
 	
    A. Deficiencies of AT-III, protein C, and protein S.
    B. Deficiencies of AT-III, heparin cofactor II, and antiphospholipid antibody syndrome.
    C. Deficiencies of AT-III, heparin cofactor II, and Soulier-Boffa syndrome.
    D. Antiphospholipid antibody syndrome and Soulier-Boffa syndrome.
	A
	
	H:504
	L:640–641
	M:465
	T:285–286

37. Plasminogen activators convert:
 	
    A. Plasmin to plasminogen.
    B. Plasminogen to plasmin.
    C. Plasminogen to fibrinogen.
    D. Fibrinogen to plasminogen.
	B
	
	H:488
	L:590
	M:402
	T:282

38. Naturally occurring plasminogen activators include:
    A. Serine proteases.
    B. Serine proteases and streptokinase.
    C. Urokinase and tPA.
    D. Urokinase, streptokinase, and serine protease.
	C
	
	H:488
	L:591
	M:404
	T:282

Select the Best Answer	Answers & References
39. The thrombolytic agents are designed to: A. Convert plasminogen to plasmin, which lyse fibrin. B. Produce alpha-2-antiplasmin. C. Inhibit factors XII and XIII. D. Prevent platelet aggregation.	A H:513 L:651 M:x T:282
40. The process of fibrin degradation is called _____, which is primarily controlled by the enzyme _____. A. Fibrination, plasmin B. Fibrinolysis, plasmin C. Fibrination, protease D. Fibrinolysis, protease	B H:430 L:590 M:405 T:282
41. A 62-year-old female presents with jaundice and the following laboratory data: Peripheral blood smear: Macrocytes Platelet count = 355 × 10^9/L PT = 25 s APTT = 35 s Alanine aminotransferase (ALT/SGPT): Elevated Lactic dehydrogenase: Elevated Bilirubin: Elevated The most probable diagnosis is: A. Sterile gut syndrome. B. Congenital factor VII deficiency. C. Cirrhosis of the liver. D. Disseminated intravascular coagulation.	C H:234 L:164 M:183 T:287
42. An 18-year-old male is seen in the emergency department following a snake bite and with evidence of bleeding episodes. Laboratory data reveal the following: Peripheral blood smear: Schizocytes (schistocytes) and spherocytes Platelet count = 75 × 10^9/L PT = 18 s APTT = 52 s D-Dimer: Positive The most probable diagnosis is: A. Malabsorption syndrome. B. Vitamin K deficiency. C. Primary fibrinolysis. D. Disseminated intravascular coagulation.	D H:493 L:635 M:457 T:290−292

Select the Best Answer	Answers & References

43. The following laboratory data were obtained on a 15-year-old female with menorrhagia:
 	
    Complete blood count: Normal
    PT = 12 s
    APTT = 45 s
    Bleeding time = 16.5 min
    Platelet retention = 20%
    Platelet aggregation studies: Abnormal with ristocetin
 	
The most probable diagnosis is:
 	
A. von Willebrand's disease.
 	
B. Aspirin ingestion.
 	
C. Hemophilia A.
 	
D. Hemophilia B.
	A
	
	H:470
	
	L:630
	
	M:443
	
	T:287–289

Section Four

APPENDICES

Appendix A

Hematology Laboratory Calculations

I. Prefixes commonly used in hematology calculations
   A. Deci (d): 10^{-1} or 0.1
   B. Centi (c): 10^{-2} or 0.01
   C. Milli (m): 10^{-3} or 0.001
   D. Micro (μ): 10^{-6} or 0.000001
   E. Nano (n): 10^{-9} or 0.000000001
   F. Pico (p): 10^{-12} or 0.000000000001
   G. Femto (f): 10^{-15} or 0.000000000000001

II. Myeloid : erythroid (M : E) ratio
   A. Calculation: The ratio is calculated by dividing the total number of granulocytes and their precursors by the total number of nucleated RBCs.
   B. Example: (bone marrow differential – 300 cell count).

Myeloblasts	10
Promyelocytes	30
Myelocytes	45
Metamyelocytes	60
Band neutrophils	30
Segmented neutrophils	15
Lymphoblasts	5
Lymphocytes	30
Plasma cells	3
Monocytes	12
Rubriblasts	6
Prorubricytes	9
Rubricytes	30
Metarubricytes	15

   Total number of granulocytes = 190
   Total number of NRBCs = 60
   M : E ratio = 190 : 60 or 3.2 : 1

III. Cell counts using a Neubauer hemacytometer
   A. One must consider three factors involved in manual cell counting:
      1. Dilution of the specimen
         a. A specimen for a WBC count is often diluted using a WBC Thoma pipet. Blood may be drawn to the 0.5 mark and diluting fluid to the 11 mark for a dilution of 1 : 20, or blood may be drawn to the 1.0 mark and diluting fluid to the 11 mark for a dilution of 1 : 10.
         b. A specimen for a RBC count is often diluted using a RBC Thoma pipet. Blood may be drawn to the 0.5 mark and diluting fluid to the 101 mark for a dilution of 1 : 200, or blood may be drawn to the 1.0 mark and diluting fluid to the 101 mark for a dilution of 1 : 100.
         c. A specimen for a platelet count is often diluted using a RBC Thoma pipet. Blood may be drawn to the 0.5 mark and diluting fluid to the 101 mark for a dilution of 1 : 200, or blood may be drawn to the 1.0 mark and diluting fluid to the 101 mark for a dilution of 1 : 100.
      2. Area of the hemacytometer counted
         a. WBCs are usually counted in the four primary corner squares with a total area of 1 mm × 1 mm × 4 squares. The total area is 4 mm².
         b. RBCs are usually counted in five secondary center squares with a total area of 0.2 mm × 0.2 mm × 5 squares. The total area is 0.2 mm².
         c. Platelets are usually counted in the center primary square with a total area of 1 mm × 1 mm × 1 square. The total area is 1 mm².
      3. Depth between the hemacytometer and the cover glass: 0.1 mm

B. Calculation: Actual cell count = (CC) (DR)(AR)(HDR), where

> CC = number of cells (WBCs, RBCs, or platelets) counted
> DR = reciprocal of the dilution
> AR = reciprocal of the area counted
> HDR = reciprocal of the hemacytometer depth

C. Examples:

1. 250 WBCs are counted in the four primary corner squares of a Neubauer hemacytometer. Blood was drawn to the 1 mark and diluting fluid to the 11 mark of a WBC Thoma pipet.

> Cells counted = 250
> Dilution = 1:10; therefore the reciprocal is 10
> Area = $1 \times 1 \times 4 = 4$; therefore the reciprocal is ¼ or 0.25
> Depth = ¹⁄₁₀; therefore the reciprocal is 10

> Actual cell count = $(250)(10)(0.25)(10) = 6.3 \times 10^3/mm^3$ or $6.3 \times 10^9/L$

2. 400 RBCs are counted in the ten secondary center squares of a Neubauer hemacytometer. Blood was drawn to the 0.5 mark and diluting fluid to the 101 mark of a RBC Thoma pipet.

> Cells counted = 400
> Dilution = 1:200; therefore the reciprocal is 200
> Area = $0.2 \times 0.2 \times 10 = 0.4$; therefore the reciprocal is ¹⁄₀.₄ or 2.5
> Depth = ¹⁄₁₀; therefore the reciprocal is 10

> Actual cell count = $(400)(200)(2.5)(10) = 2.00 \times 10^6/mm^3$ or $2.00 \times 10^{12}/L$

3. 150 platelets are counted in the primary center square of both sides of a Neubauer hemacytometer. Blood was drawn to the 1 mark and diluting fluid to the 101 mark of a RBC Thoma pipet.

> Cells counted = 150
> Dilution = 1:100; therefore the reciprocal is 100
> Area = $1 \times 1 \times 2 = 2$; therefore the reciprocal is ½ or 0.5
> Depth = ¹⁄₁₀; therefore the reciprocal is 10

> Actual cell count = $(150)(100)(0.5)(10) = 75 \times 10^3/mm^3$ or $75 \times 10^9/L$

IV. Reticulocyte count

A. Calculations

1. Uncorrected count: Percentage of reticulocytes in total RBCs counted.

2. Corrected count: Uncorrected count multiplied by the patient's hematocrit divided by the mean of the normal range for hematocrit.

3. Reticulocyte production index (RPI): Corrected count divided by the maturation time of shift reticulocytes.

Hematocrit (L/L)	Maturation Time (Days)
0.45	1.0
0.35	1.5
0.25	2.0
0.15	2.5

Adapted from Hillman RS and Finch CA: *Red Cell Manual*, ed 5. Philadelphia, FA Davis Co., 1985, p. 50, with permission.

4. Absolute reticulocyte count: Total RBC count multiplied by the uncorrected percentage of reticulocytes. Report as reticulocytes $\times 10^9/L$.

B. Examples

1. A 56-year-old male has the following laboratory data:

> RBC = $2.85 \times 10^{12}/L$
> Hematocrit = 0.25 L/L (normal range for adult males: 0.40–0.54 L/L)
> Reticulocytes/1000 RBCs = 75

> Uncorrected reticulocyte count = $(75 \div 1000) \times 100 = 7.5\%$
> Corrected reticulocyte count = $7.5\% \times (0.25 \div 0.47) = 4.0\%$
> Reticulocyte production index = $4.0\% \div 2.0 = 2.0\%$
> Absolute reticulocyte count = $7.5\% \times (2.85 \times 10^{12}/L) = 0.075 \times (2.85 \times 10^{12}/L) = 0.214 \times 10^{12}/L$ or $214 \times 10^9/L$

2. A 22-year-old female has the following laboratory data:

> RBC = $3.90 \times 10^{12}/L$
> Hematocrit = 0.35 L/L (normal range for adult females: 0.36–0.48 L/L)
> Reticulocytes/1000 RBCs = 20

Uncorrected reticulocyte count =
$$(20 \div 1000) \times 100 = 2.0\%$$
Corrected reticulocyte count =
$$2.0\% \times (0.35 \div 0.42) = 1.7\%$$
Reticulocyte production index =
$$1.7\% \div 1.5 = 1.1\%$$
Absolute reticulocyte count =
$$2.0\% \times (3.90 \times 10^{12}/L) =$$
$$0.02 \times (3.90 \times 10^{12}/L) =$$
$$0.078 \times 10^{12}/L \text{ or } 78 \times 10^9/L$$

V. RBC indices
  A. Calculations
    1. Mean cell volume (MCV)

$$MCV \text{ (in fL)} = \frac{Hct \text{ (in L/L)}}{RBC/L} \text{ or}$$
$$= \frac{Hct \text{ (in \%)} \times 10}{RBC/\mu L}$$

    2. Mean cell hemoglobin (MCH)

$$MCH \text{ (in pg)} = \frac{Hb \text{ (in g/L)}}{RBC/L} \text{ or}$$
$$= \frac{Hb \text{ (in g/dL)}}{RBC/\mu L}$$

    3. Mean cell hemoglobin concentration (MCHC)

$$MCHC \text{ (in g/L)} = \frac{Hb \text{ (in g/L)}}{Hct \text{ (in L/L)}} \text{ or}$$
$$= \frac{Hb \text{ (in g/dL)}}{Hct \text{ (in \%)}}$$

  B. Examples
    1. A patient has the following laboratory data:

RBC = $2.85 \times 10^{12}/L$
Hemoglobin = 90 g/L
Hematocrit = 0.25 L/L

MCV = $0.25 \div (2.85 \times 10^{12})$
   $= 8.77 \times 10^{-14}$ L or 87.7 fL
MCH = $90 \div (2.85 \times 10^{12})$
   $= 3.16 \times 10^{-11}$ g or 31.6 pg
MCHC = $90 \div 0.25$
   $= 360$ g/L

    2. A patient has the following laboratory data:

RBC = $4.75 \times 10^{12}/L$
Hemoglobin = 130 g/L
Hematocrit = 0.45 L/L

MCV = $0.45 \div (4.75 \times 10^{12})$
   $= 9.47 \times 10^{-14}$ L or 94.7 fL

MCH = $130 \div (4.75 \times 10^{12})$
   $= 2.74 \times 10^{-11}$ g or 27.4 pg
MCHC = $130 \div 0.40$
   $= 325$ g/L

VI. Absolute differential count
  A. Calculation: The total WBC count is multiplied by the percentage of cells from the differential.
  B. Examples:
    1. A patient had the following laboratory data:

WBC = $8.0 \times 10^9/L$

Relative counts from the differential

Neutrophils (bands and segs) = 80%
Lymphocytes = 20%

Absolute number of neutrophils =
   $0.80 \times (8.0 \times 10^9) = 6.4 \times 10^9/L$
Absolute number of lymphocytes =
   $0.20 \times (8.0 \times 10^9) = 1.6 \times 10^9/L$)

    2. A patient had the following laboratory data:

WBC = $30.0 \times 10^9/L$

Relative counts from the differential

Neutrophils (bands and segs) = 80%
Lymphocytes = 20%

Absolute number of neutrophils =
   $0.80 \times (30.0 \times 10^9) = 24.0 \times 10^9/L$
Absolute number of lymphocytes =
   $0.20 \times (30.0 \times 10^9) = 6.0 \times 10^9/L$

VII. WBC corrections for nucleated RBCs
  A. Calculation:

Corrected WBC count =

$$\frac{WBC/L \times 100}{NRBC \text{ per } 100 \text{ WBCs} + 100}$$

  B. Examples:
    1. A patient has a WBC count of $24.0 \times 10^9/L$. Fifty NRBCs per 100 WBCs were seen on the differential. Calculate the corrected WBC count.

Corrected WBC =

$$\frac{(24.0 \times 10^9/L) \times 100}{50 + 100}$$

$$= 16.0 \times 10^9/L$$

    2. A newborn with hemolytic disease of the newborn has a WBC count of $18.0 \times 10^9/L$. Two hundred eighty-five NRBCs

per 100 WBCs were seen on the differential. Calculate the corrected WBC count.

Corrected WBC =

$$\frac{(18.0 \times 10^9/L) \times 100}{285 + 100}$$

$$= 4.7 \times 10^9/L$$

VIII. International normalized ratio (INR)

A. Calculation: To report prothrombin times (PTs) as INRs, the following formula is used:

INR = (patient PT in seconds ÷ PT reference mean in seconds)^{ISI}

where ISI = International Sensitivity Index supplied by the manufacturer of the PT reagent.

B. Examples:

1. A patient's PT is 20.1 seconds. The PT reference time mean is 12.5 seconds. The ISI is 1.55. Calculate the INR.

INR = $(20.1 \div 12.5)^{1.55}$ = 2.1

2. A patient's PT is 25.0 seconds. The PT reference time mean is 12.5 seconds. The ISI is 1.25. Calculate the INR.

INR = $(25.0 \div 12.5)^{1.25}$ = 2.4

IX. Blood to anticoagulant ratio adjustment

A. Calculation: Most coagulation tests use platelet-poor plasma from blood anticoagulated at a 9:1 ratio with sodium citrate. Volume adjustments must be made with specimens collected from patients with extremely high (>60%, 0.60 L/L) or extremely low (<20%, 0.20 L/L) hematocrits. The amount of anticoagulant may be adjusted using the following formula:

$C = (0.00185)(V)(100 -$ patient's hematocrit in %)

where $V =$ volume of patient's blood in milliliters and $C =$ volume of anticoagulant in milliliters.

B. Examples:

1. A patient's hematocrit is 65 percent. The laboratorian desires to collect 4.5 milliliters of blood. Calculate the amount of sodium citrate needed.

$C = (0.00185)(4.5)(100 - 65)$
$= 0.29$ mL of anticoagulant

2. A patient's hematocrit is 15 percent. The laboratorian desires to use a collection tube with 0.5 milliliter of sodium citrate. Calculate the amount of blood needed.

$0.5 = (0.00185)(V)(100 - 15)$
$V = 3.18$ mL of blood

Appendix B

Normal Ranges

ADULT REFERENCE RANGES		
Test	**Conventional Units**	**System of International Units**
Hematology		
WBC count	$4.5-11.0 \times 10^3/\mu L$	$4.5-11.0 \times 10^9/L$
RBC count	Male: $4.50-6.00 \times 10^6/\mu L$ Female: $4.00-5.50 \times 10^6/\mu L$	Male: $4.50-6.00 \times 10^{12}/L$ Female: $4.00-5.50 \times 10^{12}/L$
Hemoglobin	Male: 13.5–18.0 g/dL Female: 12.0–16.0 g/dL	Male: 135–180 g/L Female: 120–160 g/L
Hematocrit	Male: 40–54% Female: 36–48%	Male: 0.40–0.54 L/L Female: 0.36–0.48 L/L
MCV	$80-98 \ \mu m^3$	80–98 fL
MCH	27–32 pg	27–32 pg
MCHC	32–36 g/dL	320–360 g/L
RDW	11.5–14.5%	11.5–14.5%
Platelet count	$140-415 \times 10^3/\mu L$	$140-415 \times 10^9/L$
MPV	7.4–10.4 fL	7.4–10.4 fL
Percentage of neutrophils	47–68%	47–68%
Absolute number of neutrophils	$1.8-7.5 \times 10^3/\mu L$	$1.8-7.5 \times 10^9/L$
Percentage of lymphocytes	18–54%	18–54%
Absolute number of lymphocytes	$1.1-3.8 \times 10^3/\mu L$	$1.1-3.8 \times 10^9/L$
Percentage of monocytes	2–10%	2–10%
Absolute number of monocytes	$0.1-0.8 \times 10^3/\mu L$	$0.1-0.8 \times 10^9/L$
Percentage of eosinophils	1–6%	1–6%
Absolute number of eosinophils	$0.05-0.6 \times 10^3/\mu L$	$0.05-0.6 \times 10^9/L$
Percentage of basophils	0–2%	0–2%
Absolute number of basophils	$0-0.2 \times 10^3/\mu L$	$0-0.2 \times 10^9/L$
Percentage of reticulocytes	0.5–1.8%	0.5–1.8%
Absolute number of reticulocytes	$23-108 \times 10^3/\mu L$	$23-108 \times 10^9/L$
Acidified serum lysis (Ham's) test	No hemolysis	No hemolysis
Donath-Landsteiner test	Negative	Negative
Erythrocyte sedimentation rate (Westergren)	Male: <11 mm/h Female: <16 mm/h	Male: <11 mm/h Female: <16 mm/h

ADULT REFERENCE RANGES		
Test	**Conventional Units**	**System of International Units**
G6PD spot test	Fluorescence	Fluorescence
Hemoglobin A	95–98%	95–98%
Hemoglobin A_2	1.8–3.5%	1.8–3.5%
Hemoglobin F	0–2%	0–2%
Osmotic fragility	Begin hemolysis at 0.45% End hemolysis at 0.30%	Begin hemolysis at 0.45% End hemolysis at 0.30%
Sucrose hemolysis test	No hemolysis	No hemolysis
Chemistry		
Haptoglobin	35–240 mg/dL	0.35–2.4 g/L
RBC folate	150–700 ng/mL	340–1590 nmol/L
Schilling test	>8%	>8%
Serum B_{12} (RIA)	200–900 pg/mL	150–675 pmol/L
Serum ferritin	Male: 20–270 ng/mL Female: 16–150 ng/mL	Male: 20–270 μg/L Female: 16–150 μg/L
Serum folate	2–16 ng/mL	4–36 nmol/L
Serum iron	55–160 μg/dL	10–29 μmol/L
Total iron binding capacity	230–400 μg/dL	41–72 μmol/L
Transferrin saturation	20–55%	20–55%
Blood Bank		
Direct antiglobulin test	Negative	Negative
Indirect antiglobulin test	Negative	Negative
Coagulation		
Activated partial thromboplastin time	22–40 s	22–40 s
Bleeding time	2–9 min	2–9 min
Clot retraction	50–80%	0.50–0.80
D-Dimer	<0.5 μg/mL	<0.0005 g/L
Euglobulin lysis time	No clot lysis in 2 h	No clot lysis in 2 h
Fibrinogen	155–405 mg/dL	1.55–4.05 g/L
Fibrin(ogen) split products	<10 μg/mL	<0.01 g/L
Lee-White clotting time	5–15 min	5–15 min
Plasminogen	0.1–0.2 mg/mL	1–2 μm
Platelet retention	70–90%	70–90%
Protamine sulfate test	Negative	Negative
Prothrombin time	10.0–14.0 s	10.0–14.0 s
Thrombin time	8–15 s	8–15 s
Urea solubility test	Intact clot after 24 h	Intact clot after 24 h
Whole blood clot lysis	Intact clot after 24 h	Intact clot after 24 h

The above reference ranges are provided for educational purposes only and reflect values that are comparable to various literature sources. However, since normal values vary according to technique and patient population, each laboratory must establish its own reference ranges.

Appendix C

♣

Comprehensive Examination

Select the Best Answer	Answers & References
1. If one or more of the normal enzymatic steps in heme synthesis is defective, the resultant metabolic disorder is called a:	A
A. Porphyria.	H:88
B. Thalassemia.	L:84
C. Hemoglobinopathy.	M:126
D. Hemolytic anemia.	T:65
2. Hemoglobin F corresponds to which of the following globin chains?	B
A. $\alpha_2\beta_2$	H:11
B. $\alpha_2\gamma_2$	L:73
C. $\alpha_2\delta_2$	M:39
D. $\alpha_2\epsilon_2$	T:66
3. The normal M:E ratio for adults is:	C
A. 1.5:1 to 1:3.	H:49
B. 1:1.5 to 2:4.	L:377
C. 2:1 to 4:1.	M:101
D. 3:1 to 6:1.	T:356
4. A person with hereditary elliptocytosis is most likely to have:	D
A. Aplastic anemia.	H:127
B. Decreased hematopoiesis.	L:246
C. Intravascular hemolysis.	M:206–207
D. Extravascular hemolysis.	T:x
5. A hemoglobin molecule in which iron is in the ferric (Fe^{3+}) state is called:	B
A. Carboxyhemoglobin.	H:14
B. Methemoglobin.	L:67
C. Ferrihemoglobin.	M:33
D. Sulfhemoglobin.	T:68

Select the Best Answer	Answers & References
6. A nucleated RBC that contains excessive iron is called a:	D
A. Ferricyte.	H:11
B. Ferriblast.	L:78
C. Siderocyte.	M:114
D. Sideroblast.	T:380
7. A blood specimen reveals 97% hemoglobin A, 2% hemoglobin A_2, and 1% hemoglobin F. The next step is to:	C
A. Recollect the specimen.	H:10
B. Perform a Kleihauer-Betke stain.	L:73
C. Send out the report.	M:38–40
D. Quantitate hemoglobin A_2 by column chromatography.	T:67
8. Ninety percent of the ATP or glucose required by RBCs is provided by the:	D
A. Luebering-Rapoport pathway.	H:15
B. Hexose monophosphate (pentose phosphate) shunt.	L:248
C. Methemoglobin reductase pathway.	M:30
D. Embden-Meyerhof pathway.	T:71
9. Metheme is transported by:	A
A. Hemopexin.	H:18
B. Lactoferrin.	L:234
C. Transferrin.	M:48
D. Haptoglobin.	T:75
10. Codocytes (target cells) and acanthocytes may be produced by accumulation of:	D
A. Iron.	H:5
B. Protein.	L:93–94
C. Albumin.	M:28
D. Cholesterol.	T:88, 91
11. The globin chains $\alpha_2\beta_2$ correspond to hemoglobin:	A
A. A.	H:11
B. A_2.	L:73
C. F.	M:38
D. Gower 1.	T:65
12. The average life-span of a normal RBC is _____ days.	D
A. 30	H:16
B. 60	L:65
C. 90	M:25
D. 120	T:60

Select the Best Answer	Answers & References

13. Iron is transported to the RBC membrane by:
    A. Ferritin.
    B. Transferrin.
    C. Haptoglobin.
    D. Hemosiderin.
	B
	H:8
	L:78
	M:112
	T:99–100

14. The hemoglobin pigment that cannot be quantitated by the cyanmethemoglobin method is:
    A. Methemoglobin.
    B. Sulfhemoglobin.
    C. Deoxyhemoglobin.
    D. Carboxyhemoglobin.
	B
	H:14, 59
	L:109
	M:45
	T:x

15. Heinz bodies may be found when there is a defect in the:
    A. Kreb's cycle.
    B. Luebering-Rapoport pathway.
    C. Hexose monophosphate (pentose phosphate) shunt.
    D. Embden-Meyerhof pathway.
	C
	H:16
	L:68, 100
	M:33
	T:73

16. Hemoglobinemia, hemoglobinuria, and decreased haptoglobin are evidence of what kind of hemolysis (catabolism)?
    A. Anoxic
    B. Intravascular
    C. Extravascular
    D. Sequestration
	B
	H:17–18
	L:234, 236
	M:x
	T:74–75

17. Dacryocytes (teardrop cells) are associated with:
    A. Medullary hematopoiesis.
    B. Extramedullary hematopoiesis.
    C. Mechanical RBC destruction.
    D. Intrinsic RBC membrane defects.
	B
	H:23
	L:47
	M:11
	T:x

18. The blue color of the cytoplasm of immature cells is due to an abundance of:
    A. DNA.
    B. RNA.
    C. Hemoglobin.
    D. Iron.
	B
	H:29
	L:64
	M:6
	T:58

19. The predominant RBC precursor in normal adult marrow is the:
    A. Rubricyte.
    B. Rubriblast.
    C. Prorubricyte.
    D. Metarubricyte.
	A
	H:29
	L:x
	M:101
	T:356

Select the Best Answer	Answers & References

20. The main site of hematopoiesis in the fetus from the second month to the seventh month is the:
   A. Liver.
   B. Kidney.
   C. Lymph nodes.
   D. Bone marrow.
	A
	H:22
	L:47
	M:20
	T:44–45

21. Which of the following is *not* a common site of bone marrow biopsies and aspirates in adults?
   A. Sternum
   B. Tibia
   C. Anterior superior iliac crest
   D. Posterior superior iliac crest
	B
	H:45
	L:47
	M:x
	T:26

22. What is the diameter of a normal mature RBC in μm?
   A. 2–4
   B. 6–8
   C. 10–12
   D. 14–18
	B
	H:30
	L:64
	M:27
	T:60

23. The Prussian blue stain is used to identify:
   A. Heinz bodies.
   B. Cabot rings.
   C. Howell-Jolly bodies.
   D. Iron stores.
	D
	H:51
	L:387
	M:114
	T:380

24. Age, gender, and geographic altitude influence the:
   A. WBC count.
   B. Platelet count.
   C. Mean cell volume.
   D. Hemoglobin level.
	D
	H:55
	L:x
	M:86, 293
	T:x

25. The test used to determine whether RBCs are hypo- or hypersensitive to lysis is the:
   A. Fluorescent spot test.
   B. Hemoglobin electrophoresis.
   C. Shake test.
   D. Osmotic fragility test.
	D
	H:61
	L:245
	M:203
	T:365–366

26. The test used to screen for G6PD and pyruvate kinase deficiencies is the:
   A. Antiglobulin test.
   B. Hemoglobin electrophoresis.
   C. Fluorescent spot test.
   D. Reticulocyte count.
	C
	H:61
	L:250, 252
	M:216
	T:357

Select the Best Answer	Answers & References
27. An adult male with a RBC count of $5.00 \times 10^{12}/L$ is considered: A. Anemic. B. Polycythemic. C. Normal. D. Leukemic.	C H:527 L:108 M:3 T:341
28. Bone marrow cellularity is determined by comparing: A. Granulocytes and their precursors to nucleated RBCs. B. Nucleated RBCs to fat cells. C. Nucleated hematopoietic cells to granulocytes and their precursors. D. Nucleated hematopoietic cells to fat cells.	D H:49 L:374 M:102 T:356
29. Hemoglobinometry is based on the direct measurement of: A. Hemoglobin. B. Oxyhemoglobin. C. Carboxyhemoglobin. D. Cyanmethemoglobin.	D H:535 L:108–109 M:x T:341
30. The approximate ratio of hemoglobin to hematocrit is: A. 1:2. B. 2:1. C. 1:3. D. 3:1.	C H:57 L:113 M:85 T:x
31. The two parameters used to calculate the hematocrit are the: A. RBC count and MCH. B. MCV and hemoglobin. C. RBC count and MCV. D. MCV and MCH.	C H:59 L:113 M:85 T:x
32. Codocytes (target cells) and drepanocytes (sickle cells) are seen on the peripheral blood smear of a 6-month-old black male. The next step would be to perform a(n): A. Hemoglobin quantitation. B. Osmotic fragility. C. Hemoglobin electrophoresis. D. Bone marrow aspiration and biopsy.	C H:60 L:188 M:132 T:111
33. The best indicator of the status of storage iron is the level of serum: A. Iron. B. Ferritin. C. Protoporphyrin. D. Iron binding capacity.	B H:62 L:173 M:114 T:x

Select the Best Answer	Answers & References

34. Spherocytosis will cause the osmotic fragility test to be:
    A. Normal.
    B. Decreased.
    C. Increased.
    D. Variable.
	C
	H:61
	L:245
	M:205
	T:367

35. A patient has a RDW of 18.2%. What should be seen on the peripheral smear?
    A. Anisocytosis
    B. Poikilocytosis
    C. Acanthocytosis
    D. Schistocytosis
	A
	H:57
	L:92
	M:88
	T:315

36. A reticulocyte count is ordered on a patient with a hemolytic crisis due to G6PD deficiency. What feature may also be present?
    A. Rouleaux
    B. Heinz bodies
    C. Howell-Jolly bodies
    D. Stomatocytes
	B
	H:71
	L:100
	M:213
	T:107

37. Pappenheimer bodies may be seen when a patient has:
    A. Abetalipoproteinemia.
    B. Sideroblastic anemia.
    C. Iron deficiency anemia.
    D. Paroxysmal cold hemoglobinuria.
	B
	H:71
	L:98–99
	M:123
	T:93, 101

38. A 30-year-old female who works at a battery manufacturing company goes to the physician for a routine physical examination. The peripheral blood smear shows moderate amounts of basophilic stippling. The patient may be in the initial stages of:
    A. Multiple myeloma.
    B. Myeloid metaplasia.
    C. Leukemoid reaction.
    D. Lead intoxication.
	D
	H:71
	L:98
	M:98
	T:92

39. Spherocytes may be seen in hereditary spherocytosis and:
    A. Liver disease.
    B. Severe burns.
    C. Porphyria.
    D. Aminase deficiency.
	B
	H:68
	L:x
	M:94
	T:91

40. Nuclear remnants of DNA are called:
    A. Cabot rings.
    B. Heinz bodies.
    C. Howell-Jolly bodies.
    D. Auer rods.
	C
	H:71
	L:98
	M:98
	T:92

Select the Best Answer	Answers & References

41. Intracellular aggregates of RNA are called:
   A. Cabot rings.
   B. Howell-Jolly bodies.
   C. Toxic granulation.
   D. Basophilic stippling.
	D
	H:71
	L:98
	M:97
	T:92

42. Heinz bodies are composed of:
   A. Iron.
   B. DNA.
   C. RNA.
   D. Denatured hemoglobin.
	D
	H:71
	L:100
	M:98
	T:92

43. Severe bacterial infections may cause all the following *except*:
   A. Cabot rings.
   B. Döhle bodies.
   C. Cytoplasmic vacuoles.
   D. Toxic granulation.
	A
	H:72
	L:339
	M:258
	T:50,145−146

44. A 54-year-old male presents with a blood alcohol level of 265 mg/dL. The peripheral blood smear shows codocytes (target cells). The osmotic fragility test should be:
   A. Normal.
   B. Decreased.
   C. Increased.
   D. Variable.
	B
	H:68
	L:245
	M:205
	T:367

45. RBC agglutination will cause falsely elevated:
   A. RBC counts.
   B. Hemoglobin levels.
   C. Mean cell volumes.
   D. Platelet counts.
	C
	H:x
	L:89
	M:99−100
	T:x

46. An aid for dealing with RBC agglutination in a laboratory specimen is to:
   A. Remove the plasma.
   B. Warm the specimen.
   C. Recollect the specimen.
   D. Replace the plasma with saline.
	B
	H:70
	L:89
	M:100
	T:x

47. In most patients, the major source of daily iron is:
   A. Dietary iron.
   B. Elemental iron.
   C. Supplemental iron.
   D. Senescent RBCs.
	D
	H:81
	L:77−78
	M:110
	T:99−100

Select the Best Answer	Answers & References

48. A 45-year-old female presents with general fatigue and the following laboratory results:

Laboratory Test	Normal Range	Patient
Hemoglobin (g/L)	120–160	81
Serum iron (μg/dL)	55–160	38
Total iron-binding capacity (TIBC) (μg/dL)	230–400	275
Transferrin saturation (%)	20–55	12
Serum ferritin (ng/mL)	16–150	155

    The most likely diagnosis is:

    A. Iron deficiency anemia.

    B. Sideroblastic anemia.

    C. Anemia of chronic disease (inflammation).

    D. Anemia of unknown origin.

C

H:85

L:178

M:125

T:102

49. The most common cause of anemia in infancy, childhood, and pregnancy is:

    A. Sickle cell disease.

    B. Gastrointestinal bleeding.

    C. Iron deficiency.

    D. Inflammation.

C

H:79

L:174

M:116

T:x

50. The presence of Cabot rings and Howell-Jolly bodies on a peripheral blood smear are most indicative of:

    A. Congenital non-spherocytic hemolytic anemia.

    B. Sideroblastic anemia.

    C. Megaloblastic anemia.

    D. An iron metabolism defect.

C

H:99

L:157–158

M:168

T:92–93

51. An otherwise healthy, 23-year-old white male recently returned from Peace Corps work in Africa. He presents with intermittent chills and fever. A Wright-Giemsa stain should be evaluated for:

    A. Malaria.

    B. Leishmania.

    C. G6PD deficiency.

    D. Spherocytes.

A

H:212

L:x

M:x

T:93–94

Select the Best Answer	Answers & References
52. Intrinsic factor and vitamin B_{12} are given to a patient with a low Schilling test. If the Schilling test remains abnormal, the most likely diagnosis is:	C
A. Pernicious anemia.	H:103
B. Vitamin B_{12} deficiency.	L:161
C. Malabsorption of vitamin B_{12}.	M:178
D. Deficiency of intrinsic factor.	T:x
53. An aid for dealing with rouleaux in a laboratory specimen is to:	D
A. Remove the plasma.	H:71
B. Warm the specimen.	L:x
C. Recollect the specimen.	M:99
D. Replace the plasma with saline.	T:x
54. An autosomal recessive disorder that results in aplastic anemia as well as skeletal abnormalities and renal dysfunction is:	C
A. Aplastic anemia.	H:110
B. Megaloblastic anemia.	L:144
C. Fanconi's anemia.	M:189
D. Pure RBC aplasia.	T:98
55. A patient presents with aplastic anemia. Which of the following statements obtained during the clinical history is useful in making a diagnosis?	A
A. She recently has taken chloramphenicol for an infection.	H:109
B. She is a secretary at a local hospital.	L:139
C. A family member has hemophilia A.	M:187
D. She has intentionally lost 10 pounds in the last 2 months.	T:98
56. A common treatment for intrinsic RBC membrane disorders such as hereditary spherocytosis is:	A
A. Splenectomy.	H:124
B. Therapeutic phlebotomy.	L:247
C. Transfusion of packed RBCs.	M:206
D. Supportive therapy.	T:106
57. A defect in the hexose monophosphate (pentose phosphate) shunt may be associated with a deficiency of:	C
A. Pyruvate kinase.	H:135
B. Phosphate kinase.	L:248
C. G6PD.	M:x
D. 2,3-DPG.	T:72

Select the Best Answer	Answers & References

58. The treatment of choice for severe aplastic anemia in a 35-year-old patient is:
    A. Supportive therapy.
    B. Immunosuppressive therapy.
    C. Massive blood transfusions.
    D. Bone marrow transplantation.
	D
	H:111
	L:141–142
	M:186–187
	T:98

59. Favism may be associated with a deficiency of:
    A. 2,3-DPG.
    B. G6PD.
    C. Pyruvate kinase.
    D. Fetal hemoglobin.
	B
	H:136
	L:252
	M:x
	T:107

60. In which hemoglobinopathy is the most severe anemia seen?
    A. AS
    B. SC
    C. CC
    D. SS
	D
	H:147
	L:197
	M:137, 141–143
	T:110–111

61. The majority of hemoglobinopathies are caused by:
    A. A defect in iron metabolism.
    B. Decreased production of iron.
    C. Defective synthesis of the heme molecule.
    D. An amino acid substitution in the beta globin chain.
	D
	H:143
	L:187
	M:131
	T:x

62. The possible genotype(s) of offspring from a male whose genotype is AS and a female whose genotype is AS is (are):
    A. 100% AS.
    B. 50% AA and 50% AS.
    C. 33.3% AS, 33.3% AA, and 33.3% SS.
    D. 50% AS, 25% AA, and 25% SS.
	D
	H:143
	L:187
	M:x
	T:44

Select the Best Answer	Answers & References

63. Interpret the following laboratory data, which were obtained from a 53-year-old white male.

Laboratory Test	Normal Range	Patient
Hemoglobin (g/L)	135–180	63
MCV (fL)	80–98	113.4
MCH (pg)	27–32	38.6
MCHC (g/L)	320–360	334
RDW (%)	11.5–14.5	15.1
RBC morphology	Normocytic, normochromic	Oval macrocytes Howell-Jolly bodies Anisocytosis Poikilocytosis
Reticulocyte count (%)	0.5–1.8	1.6
Serum B_{12} (pg/mL)	200–900	63
Serum folate (ng/mL)	2–16	11
RBC folate (ng/mL)	150–700	513
Anti-IF antibodies	Negative	Positive
Schilling test (% excretion)	>8	4

The most likely diagnosis is:

A. Folate deficiency.

B. Malabsorption syndrome.

C. Reticulocytosis.

D. Pernicious anemia.

D

H:101–104

L:161

M:178

T:104

64. The RBC membrane is a(n):

A. Impermeable lipid membrane surface.

B. Permeable glycoprotein cytoplasmic membrane.

C. Semi-permeable lipid bi-layer.

D. Hypopermeable lipoprotein cytoskeleton.

C

H:4

L:65

M:28

T:33

65. The purpose of the cationic pumps in the RBC is to:

A. Actively transport sodium out of the cell and calcium into the cell.

B. Actively transport sodium out of the cell and potassium into the cell.

C. Passively transport water into the cell and chloride out of the cell.

D. Passively transport chloride into the cell and bicarbonate out of the cell.

B

H:7

L:66

M:x

T:34

Select the Best Answer	Answers & References
66. The erythrocyte sedimentation rate is:	D
A. Useful in evaluating anemias.	H:532–534
B. Decreased in inflammatory disorders.	L:117–120
C. Stable under adverse environmental conditions.	M:x
D. An indicator of occult disease.	T:352–353
67. Evidence indicates that the cause of pernicious anemia is:	C
A. Excessive radiation.	H:97
B. Overexposure to certain drugs.	L:160
C. Autoantibodies to parietal cells.	M:177
D. Chronic gastric ulcers.	T:104
68. Beta-thalassemia is manifested:	C
A. In utero.	H:167
B. At birth.	L:220
C. Several months after birth.	M:151
D. In adulthood.	T:112
69. Hemoglobin electrophoresis on a newborn reveals primarily hemoglobins Bart's and H. The infant has:	D
A. No hemoglobinopathy.	H:169–170
B. Sickle cell disease.	L:217–218
C. Beta-thalassemia.	M:159
D. Alpha-thalassemia.	T:112
70. The RBC with a slit-like central pallor is called a:	D
A. Schizocyte (schistocyte).	H:69
B. Spherocyte.	L:94
C. Xerocyte.	M:94
D. Stomatocyte.	T:91
71. Beta-thalassemia differs from alpha-thalassemia in that it has a(n):	A
A. Elevated A_2 level.	H:180
B. Normal serum iron.	L:225
C. Elevated TIBC.	M:150, 159
D. Decreased ferritin.	T:112
72. The Kleihauer-Betke acid elution test demonstrates hemoglobin:	C
A. A_2.	H:172
B. C.	L:227
C. F.	M:133
D. S.	T:69

Select the Best Answer	Answers & References
73. If a patient who has iron deficiency anemia receives blood transfusions from healthy adults, the peripheral blood smear most likely will show: A. Polychromasia. B. Reticulocytes. C. Anisocytosis. D. Poikilocytosis.	C H:66 L:91 M:92 T:x
74. When valine is substituted for glutamic acid in the sixth position of the beta globin chain, the hemoglobin is known as hemoglobin: A. C. B. D. C. F. D. S.	D H:144–145 L:186–187 M:136 T:110
75. A patient has a positive acidified serum lysis (Ham's) test and decreased acetylcholinesterase. The likely diagnosis is: A. HEMPAS. B. Paroxysmal nocturnal hemoglobinuria. C. Hereditary spherocytosis. D. Mucopolysaccharidosis.	B H:186 L:263–264 M:210–211 T:109, 354
76. To ensure complement is present in a specimen for the acidified serum lysis (Ham's) test, the specimen must be: A. Fresh. B. Refrigerated until needed. C. Frozen until needed. D. Collected only in a heparinized tube.	A H:186–187 L:264 M:x T:x
77. A screening test for paroxysmal nocturnal hemoglobinuria is the: A. Sugar water test. B. Plasma hemoglobin. C. Spot fluorescence test. D. Acidified serum lysis (Ham's) test.	A H:186 L:263 M:211 T:367
78. RBCs in patients with paroxysmal nocturnal hemoglobinuria are: A. Hypersensitive to complement. B. Hyperchromic. C. Hypochromic. D. Normal.	A H:183 L:262 M:210 T:109

Select the Best Answer	Answers & References

79. The fetomaternal incompatibility most commonly associated with hemolytic disease of the newborn is due to which system?
 	
  A. ABO
  B. Kidd
  C. Duffy
  D. Rh
	A
	H:198
	L:271
	M:247
	T:119

80. A newborn infant is diagnosed with hemolytic disease of the newborn. Which of the following will probably have to be re-calculated to produce a correct result?
 	
  A. Hemoglobin
  B. Hematocrit
  C. RBC count
  D. WBC count
	D
	H:198, 547
	L:270, 328
	M:x
	T:118, 347

81. During an acute intravascular hemolytic episode, which of the following would be decreased?
 	
  A. Haptoglobin
  B. Urine hemoglobin
  C. Urine hemosiderin
  D. Plasma hemoglobin
	A
	H:196–197
	L:234
	M:47
	T:75

82. The following results were obtained on a 10-year-old black female with a recent history of viral pneumonia.	

Laboratory Test	Normal Range	Patient
Urine hemoglobin	Negative	Positive
Urine microscopic	Few cellular elements	1–2 hyaline casts 2–5 WBCs
Hemoglobin (g/L)	135–180	102
Direct antiglobulin test	Negative	Positive
Antibody screen	Negative	Positive
Antibody panel	Negative	Anti-P

The likely diagnosis is:
  A. Paroxysmal cold hemoglobinuria.
  B. Sickle cell anemia.
  C. Paroxysmal nocturnal hemoglobinuria.
  D. Iron deficiency.
	A
	H:206
	L:274
	M:241
	T:x

Select the Best Answer	Answers & References

83. The following laboratory data were obtained during evaluation of jaundice in a newborn.

Laboratory Test	Normal Range	Patient
Peripheral blood smear (newborn)	Normocytic, normochromic	Moderate spherocytosis and anisocytosis
Direct antiglobulin test (newborn)	Negative	Weakly positive
Antibody screen (newborn)	Negative	Negative
Group and type (newborn)		A positive
Group and type (mother)		O negative

The most likely cause of jaundice is incompatibility of which group?

A. Rh

B. Lewis

C. ABO

D. Kell

C

H:198–199

L:270

M:246–248

T:119

84. The Donath-Landsteiner antibody is associated with:

A. *Plasmodium* infections.

B. Infectious mononucleosis.

C. Paroxysmal cold hemoglobinuria.

D. Paroxysmal nocturnal hemoglobinuria.

C

H:206

L:274

M:241

T:356

85. Interpret the following cellulose acetate hemoglobin electrophoresis (pH 8.4).

The most likely diagnosis is:

A. Alpha-thalassemia.

B. Beta-thalassemia.

C. Sickle cell trait.

D. Sickle cell disease.

C

H:151

L:193

M:133

T:70

Select the Best Answer	Answers & References

86. The medium usually used for hemoglobin electrophoresis is:
  A. Citrate agar at an acid pH.
  B. Citrate agar at an alkaline pH.
  C. Cellulose acetate at an acid pH.
  D. Cellulose acetate at an alkaline pH.
	D
	H:536
	L:191–192
	M:132
	T:69

87. The anticoagulant that should be used to collect a specimen for an osmotic fragility test is:
  A. EDTA.
  B. Heparin.
  C. Sodium citrate.
  D. Sodium oxalate.
	B
	H:542
	L:245
	M:x
	T:366

88. A 53-year-old female with lupus presents with an elevated BUN and creatinine and is anemic. The most likely cause of the anemia is:
  A. Iron deficiency.
  B. Gastrointestinal bleeding.
  C. Renal failure with hemoglobinuria.
  D. Decreased production of erythropoietin.
	D
	H:233
	L:147
	M:35
	T:x

89. RBCs that appear like stacks of coins are referred to as:
  A. Rouleaux.
  B. Agglutination.
  C. Cryoglobulinemia.
  D. Macroglobulinemia.
	A
	H:369
	L:89
	M:99
	T:93

90. A 26-year-old black male was trapped in a burning building. When he arrives at the emergency department, his hemoglobin is 141 g/L, and the following cells are seen on the peripheral smear.	

The most likely cause of the above cells is:
  A. Burns.
  B. Sickle cell trait.
  C. Sickle cell disease.
  D. Hereditary spherocytosis.
	A
	H:68
	L:x
	M:94
	T:91

Select the Best Answer	Answers & References

91. In the osmotic fragility test, hemolysis normally begins at ——————— NaCl and ends at ——————— NaCl.
   A. 0.45%, 0.30%
   B. 0.30%, 0.45%
   C. 0.65%, 0.20%
   D. 0.20%, 0.65%
	A
	H:542
	L:245
	M:205
	T:366

92. The best test to determine whether there has been in vivo mixing of fetal and maternal blood is the:
   A. Acid phosphatase.
   B. Alkali denaturation.
   C. CBC with differential.
   D. Hemoglobin electrophoresis.
	B
	H:178
	L:194
	M:133
	T:69

93. RBC size and shape and serum immunoglobulin levels affect the:
   A. RBC count.
   B. Clotting time.
   C. Bleeding time.
   D. Erythrocyte sedimentation rate.
	D
	H:532
	L:118
	M:x
	T:352

94. Tourniquet stasis may cause a falsely:
   A. Elevated hematocrit.
   B. Decreased hematocrit.
   C. Elevated platelet count.
   D. Decreased platelet count.
	A
	H:534
	L:112
	M:x
	T:348

95. Normal cerebrospinal fluid contains:
   A. Neither RBCs nor WBCs.
   B. RBCs but not WBCs.
   C. WBCs but not RBCs.
   D. Both WBCs and RBCs.
	C
	H:x
	L:397
	M:x
	T:407

96. Which of the following is *not* a major type of leukocyte found in peripheral blood?
   A. Neutrophil
   B. Lymphocyte
   C. Monocyte
   D. Histiocyte
	D
	H:241
	L:289
	M:52
	T:344

Select the Best Answer	Answers & References
97. The following cytograms from the Technicon H*l cell counter is suggestive of: A. Monocytosis. B. Eosinophilia. C. Neutrophilia. D. Lymphocytosis. PEROX BASO	B H:559 L:506 M:x T:319–320
98. An autosomal recessive disorder that manifests itself with large lysosomal inclusions in all types of leukocytes, recurrent infections, and albinism is: A. Chédiak-Higashi disease. B. Pelger-Huët anomaly. C. May-Hegglin anomaly. D. Alder-Reilly anomaly.	A H:249 L:358 M:260 T:146
99. The inclusions in which of the following disorders may be confused with Döhle bodies? A. Chédiak-Higashi disease B. Pelger-Huët anomaly C. May-Hegglin anomaly D. Alder-Reilly anomaly	C H:252 L:357 M:260 T:146

Select the Best Answer	Answers & References

100. A CBC ordered during a routine physical examination on a male with no complaints revealed the following data:

Laboratory Test	Normal Range	Patient
WBC ($\times 10^9$/L)	4.5–11.0	6.6
RBC ($\times 10^{12}$/L)	4.5–6.0	4.57
Hemoglobin (g/L)	135–180	142
Hematocrit (L/L)	0.40–0.54	0.43
WBC differential		
Band neutrophils (%)	3–7	35
Bi-lobed neutrophils (%)	Not established	20
Segmented neutrophils (%)	47–68	5
Lymphocytes (%)	18–54	35
Monocytes (%)	2–10	5

The results are probably due to:

A. Chédiak-Higashi disease.

B. Pelger-Huët anomaly.

C. Leukemoid reaction.

D. Acute myelocytic leukemia.

B

H:252

L:356

M:259

T:146

101. Mucopolysaccharidosis associated with large, dark-staining, coarse cytoplasmic granules in leukocytes is consistent with:

A. Chédiak-Higashi disease.

B. Job's syndrome.

C. May-Hegglin anomaly.

D. Alder-Reilly anomaly.

D

H:252

L:357

M:259

T:146

102. Congenital pancytopenia (aplastic anemia) is found in:

A. Job's syndrome.

B. Pelger-Huët anomaly.

C. Chédiak-Higashi disease.

D. Fanconi's anemia.

D

H:110

L:144

M:189

T:98

103. A patient presents with a presumptive diagnosis of lupus erythematosus; however, the LE preparation is negative. The test that should be performed next is the:

A. Acidified serum lysis (Ham's).

B. Rapid plasmin reagent.

C. Antinuclear antibody.

D. Erythrocyte sedimentation rate.

C

H:x

L:333

M:x

T:178

Select the Best Answer	Answers & References

104. A 63-year-old white male presents with a chief complaint of bone pain. The peripheral blood smear reveals rouleaux. Which of the following is *not* expected to be seen considering the preliminary diagnosis?
  A. Plasma cells
  B. Monocytosis
  C. Urinary Bence Jones proteins
  D. Elevated erythrocyte sedimentation rate
	B
	H:374–376
	L:475–478
	M:360–362
	T:217

105. A 54-year-old white male presents with fatigue and lymphadenopathy. Chronic lymphocytic leukemia is suspected. Which of the following is *not* normally helpful in making a more definitive diagnosis?
  A. Lymph node biopsy
  B. Bone marrow biopsy
  C. Periodic acid-Schiff stain
  D. Leukocyte alkaline phosphatase stain
	D
	H:317–318
	L:456–457
	M:358–360
	T:228

106. Parasitic infections and allergies often cause:
  A. Basophilia.
  B. Eosinophilia.
  C. Monocytosis.
  D. Lymphocytosis.
	B
	H:x
	L:341–342
	M:261
	T:144

107. Patients with AIDS have significantly decreased numbers of helper cells known as:
  A. Neutrophils.
  B. Monocytes.
  C. CD4 cells.
  D. CD8 cells.
	C
	H:367
	L:x
	M:x
	T:175

108. Myeloperoxidase is *not* present in:
  A. Neutrophils.
  B. Eosinophils.
  C. Lymphocytes.
  D. Monocytes.
	C
	H:273
	L:x
	M:317
	T:202

109. Which of the following stains is specific for phospholipids?
  A. Sudan black B
  B. Myeloperoxidase
  C. Periodic acid-Schiff
  D. Specific esterase
	A
	H:273
	L:386
	M:318
	T:201–202

110. A large cell with voluminous, dark-blue cytoplasm that indents when it contacts RBCs is called a:
  A. Lymphocyte.
  B. Variant (reactive) lymphocyte.
  C. Monocyte.
  D. Myeloblast.
	B
	H:36
	L:291
	M:68
	T:158

Select the Best Answer	Answers & References
111. The diagnosis of erythroleukemia is aided by a positive: A. Myeloperoxidase. B. Sudan black B. C. Periodic acid-Schiff. D. Non-specific esterase.	C H:274 L:385–386 M:336 T:203
112. The marginating pool of neutrophils is located: A. In the kidneys. B. In the tissues. C. Next to the marrow sinuses. D. On the blood vessel walls.	D H:30 L:294 M:x T:130
113. T lymphocytes mature in the: A. Thyroid. B. Thymus. C. Bone marrow. D. Lymph nodes.	B H:35 L:51 M:16 T:154
114. Plasma cells originate from: A. B lymphocytes. B. T lymphocytes. C. Lymphocytes. D. Monocytes.	A H:36 L:305 M:72 T:162
115. A large cell having abundant cytoplasm with ground-glass appearance and a nucleus with a lacy pattern is called a: A. Lymphocyte. B. Monocyte. C. Variant lymphocyte. D. Plasma cell.	B H:35 L:291 M:62 T:133
116. Acute lymphoblastic leukemia type L1 is found: A. Most frequently in pediatric patients. B. Most frequently in adult patients. C. Most frequently in geriatric patients. D. Equally in all patients.	A H:287 L:450 M:339 T:198
117. Surface markers may be used to identify: A. Only cell type. B. Only development stage. C. Both cell type and development stage. D. Only monoclonal proteins.	C H:275 L:528 M:71 T:160

Select the Best Answer	Answers & References
118. High levels of terminal deoxynucleotidyl transferase are found in:	C
A. Myeloblasts.	H:276
B. Monoblasts.	L:389
C. Lymphoblasts.	M:342
D. Rubriblasts.	T:160
119. The occurrence of the Philadelphia chromosome in CML is an indicator of:	D
A. Leukemic meningitis.	H:331
B. Spontaneous remission.	L:437
C. Worse prognosis and response to therapy.	M:281
D. Better prognosis and response to therapy.	T:229
120. A patient's bone marrow shows 27% blasts with Auer rods, and he has peripheral pancytopenia. The most likely diagnosis is:	D
A. Refractory anemia.	H:300
B. Refractory anemia with ringed sideroblasts.	L:414
C. Refractory anemia with excess blasts.	M:306
D. Refractory anemia with excess blasts in transformation.	T:249
121. The technique used by Technicon hematology instrumentation for leukocyte differential analysis includes:	B
A. Volume sizing, basophilic lobularity, and cytochemistry.	H:549–551
B. Optical flow cytometry, cytochemistry, and light scatter.	L:517
C. Cytochemistry, cell conductivity, and basophilic lobularity.	M:x
D. Volume sizing, cell conductivity, and light scatter.	T:313
122. Smudge cells are seen commonly in:	B
A. ALL.	H:312
B. CLL.	L:327
C. AML.	M:358
D. CML.	T:158
123. Which of the following is consistent with leukemoid reaction?	B
A. Toxic granulation, vacuoles, and eosinophilia	H:332
B. Toxic granulation, vacuoles, and Döhle bodies	L:x
C. Marked eosinophilia, marked basophilia, and toxic granulation	M:284
D. Marked eosinophilia, marked basophilia, and giant bizarre nuclei	T:x

Select the Best Answer	Answers & References

124. Interpret the following laboratory data.

Laboratory Test	Normal Range	Patient
Patient data		57-year-old male with fatigue for 6 months
WBC ($\times 10^9$/L)	4.5–11.0	4.1
Hemoglobin (g/L)	135–180	101
Platelet count ($\times 10^9$/L)	140–415	97
WBC differential % Blasts % Promyelocytes % Myelocytes % Metamyelocytes % Band neutrophils % Segmented neutrophils % Lymphocytes % Monocytes	0 0 0 0 2–6 50–70 20–44 2–9	2 1 1 0 5 18 66 7
Comments on peripheral blood film	Normocytic, normochromic	14 NRBCs Pseudo-Pelger cells seen
Comments on bone marrow preparation	Normocellular	Marked erythroid hyperplasia and ringed sideroblasts
Cytochemical stains	Varies with the cell line	Positive for periodic acid-Schiff
Cell markers	Varies with the cell line	Negative for CD 14, CD 10 (CALLA), CD 19, and HLA-DR

The most likely diagnosis is:

A. Refractory anemia.

B. Refractory anemia with ringed sideroblasts.

C. Chronic myelomonocytic leukemia.

D. Erythroleukemia.

D
H:281
L:426
M:335–336
T:197, 203

125. The function of the T lymphocyte is to:

A. Produce immune globulins.

B. Interact with antibody to destroy antibody-coated targets.

C. Phagocytize bacteria and cellular debris.

D. Participate in cellular immunity.

D
H:24
L:308
M:69
T:158

126. An elevated LAP score is usually:

A. Found in leukemoid reaction and CML.

B. Found in leukemoid reaction but not CML.

C. Found in CML but not leukemoid reaction.

D. Not found in either leukemoid reaction or CML.

B
H:332
L:384
M:254
T:229

Select the Best Answer	Answers & References
127. A positive tartrate-resistant acid phosphatase stain may aid in diagnosing: A. ALL. B. CLL. C. Hairy cell leukemia. D. Kaposi's sarcoma.	C H:323 L:384 M:360 T:204
128. A normal RBC mass is usually found in: A. Polycythemia vera. B. Secondary polycythemia. C. Relative polycythemia. D. All the above.	C H:347 L:432–434 M:295 T:58
129. The following scattergram from a Coulter cell counter is suggestive of: A. Monocytosis. B. Eosinophilia. C. Lymphocytosis. D. Thrombocytosis.	A H:558 L:523 M:x T:x

WBC

VOLUME

DF 1

130. A 28-year-old black male presents in the emergency department with severe vomiting and diarrhea. Laboratory data reveal elevated WBC, RBC, and platelet counts. The likely cause of the abnormality is: A. Polycythemia vera. B. Instrument malfunction. C. Pulmonary insufficiency. D. Dehydration.	D H:356–357 L:434 M:295 T:x

Select the Best Answer	Answers & References
131. The preferred primary treatment in polycythemia vera is: A. Plateletpheresis. B. Phlebotomy. C. Plasmapheresis. D. Anticoagulation therapy.	B H:353 L:434 M:292 T:232
132. The primary treatments of essential thrombocythemia include all the following *except*: A. Aspirin therapy. B. Chemotherapy. C. Phlebotomy. D. Plateletpheresis.	C H:359 L:442 M:298 T:236–237
133. Which of the following is *not* a class of immunoglobulins? A. IgA B. IgC C. IgD D. IgE	B H:367 L:475 M:73 T:x
134. Intracellular aggregates of immunoglobulins are called: A. Howell-Jolly bodies. B. Russell bodies. C. Heinz bodies. D. Pappenheimer bodies.	B H:375 L:311 M:73 T:163
135. The best test for determining whether a monoclonal protein is present is: A. Serum protein electrophoresis. B. Urine electrophoresis. C. Quantitative immunoglobulin assay. D. Qualitative immunoglobulin assay.	A H:372 L:476 M:x T:217
136. Hypogammaglobulinemia is characterized by an absence of a peak after the _____ peak. A. Albumin B. Alpha-1 C. Beta D. Gamma	C H:371 L:476 M:x T:218
137. The Reed-Sternberg cell is characteristic of which lymphoma? A. B-cell B. T-cell C. Hodgkin's D. Burkitt's	C H:385 L:463 M:346 T:216

Select the Best Answer	Answers & References
138. Patients with mucopolysaccharidoses may exhibit which of the following in the peripheral blood?	D
A. Auer rods	H:408
B. Heinz bodies	L:360
C. Russell bodies	M:259
D. Alder-Reilly bodies	T:146
139. The substances that are vital for the production and proliferation of stem cells are called:	D
A. Growth hormones.	H:242
B. Stem cell factors.	L:50
C. Cell substance factors.	M:23
D. Colony-stimulating factors.	T:129
140. On the cells' surfaces, specific proteins that distinguish one cell line from another are called:	C
A. Flow cytometric analytes.	H:275
B. Light scatter proteins.	L:528
C. Cell markers.	M:x
D. Cytochemical receptors.	T:160
141. Which of the following is *not* true?	A
A. Neutrophils exchange freely between blood and tissues.	H:242
B. Neutrophils exchange freely between marginating and circulating pools.	L:294
	M:55
C. The circulating half-life of neutrophils is approximately 7–10 hours.	T:130–131
D. Neutrophils can be stored in the bone marrow until they are released into the peripheral blood.	
142. The term "left shift" commonly refers to:	D
A. Leukocytosis.	H:243
B. Immature monocytes.	L:337
C. Immature lymphocytes.	M:253
D. Immature granulocytes.	T:137
143. A significant left shift is most likely to occur in:	B
A. Viral infections.	H:243
B. Bacterial infections.	L:337
C. Parasitic infections.	M:253
D. All infections.	T:x

Select the Best Answer	Answers & References
144. The plasma proteins necessary for the efficient phagocytosis of most pathologic microorganisms are called: A. Vesicles. B. Opsonins. C. Lysosomes. D. Lipoproteins.	B H:244 L:297 M:64 T:135
145. Hypersegmentation of neutrophils is usually defined as more than how many segments? A. Two B. Four C. Six D. Eight	C H:99 L:357 M:168 T:146
146. Interpret the following laboratory data.	

Laboratory Test	Patient
Patient data	19-year-old male
CBC	WBC: normal with 90% reactive lymphocytes
Heterophile antibody test	Positive
EBV antibody test	1:512
CMV antibody test	Negative
Liver enzymes	Normal

	Answers & References
The most likely diagnosis is: A. Infectious mononucleosis without liver involvement. B. Infectious mononucleosis with liver involvement. C. CMV mononucleosis without liver involvement. D. CMV mononucleosis with liver involvement.	A H:262–263 L:352–353 M:267–270 T:170–171

147. Interpret the following laboratory data.

Laboratory Test	Patient
Platelet count	↓
RBC count	↓
WBC count	↑ with monocytosis
% Blasts in peripheral blood	3
% Blasts in bone marrow	17
% Ringed sideroblasts in bone marrow	8
Chromosomal abnormality	12q⁻

Select the Best Answer	Answers & References
The most likely diagnosis is: A. Refractory anemia. B. Refractory anemia with ringed sideroblasts. C. Refractory anemia with excess blasts. D. Chronic myelomonocytic leukemia.	D H:295–300 L:412–414 M:305–308 T:249
148. The average life-span of a circulating platelet is how many days? A. 1–3 B. 9–12 C. 30–45 D. 60–90	B H:417 L:663 M:368 T:271
149. The metabolic region of platelets is in which zone? A. Organelle B. Peripheral C. Sol-gel D. Ultrastructural	A H:418 L:660 M:370 T:x
150. Platelet adhesion is dependent upon the presence of: A. Calcium. B. Thrombin. C. Fibrinogen. D. von Willebrand factor.	D H:421 L:689 M:372 T:272
151. The extrinsic pathway is monitored by the: A. Prothrombin time. B. Thrombin time. C. Activated partial thromboplastin time. D. Factor assay.	A H:428 L:609 M:408 T:283
152. Fibrinolysis is regulated by: A. Fibrinogen. B. Plasmin. C. Protease. D. Thrombin.	B H:430 L:635 M:402 T:282
153. An elevated PT and normal APTT is consistent with a deficiency of factor: A. II. B. V. C. VII. D. X.	C H:481 L:613 M:450 T:392

Select the Best Answer	Answers & References
154. A patient with a deficiency of factor XIII usually presents with a(n): A. Elevated PT and APTT. B. Elevated PT and normal APTT. C. Normal PT and elevated APTT. D. Normal PT and APTT.	D H:481 L:633 M:450 T:x
155. A prolonged thrombin time may be seen in a patient with a deficiency of factor: A. I. B. II. C. V. D. VII.	A H:597–598 L:613 M:450 T:283
156. An abnormal urea solubility test may indicate: A. A quantitative platelet defect. B. A qualitative platelet defect. C. A deficiency of factor XIII. D. Hemophilia A.	C H:477 L:633 M:413 T:x
157. Decreased aggregation with ristocetin is often found in patients with: A. Hemophilia A. B. Hemophilia B. C. von Willebrand's disease. D. Bernard-Soulier syndrome.	C H:470 L:630 M:443 T:289
158. A patient's plasma produces an elevated PT and APTT and does *not* produce a normal PT and APTT when mixed with normal plasma. The most likely cause is: A. Procedural error. B. Prekallikrein deficiency. C. Factor inhibitors. D. von Willebrand's disease.	C H:607 L:615 M:459–460 T:292
159. A deficiency of which factor is associated with an asymptomatic presentation? A. I B. II C. XII D. XIII	C H:465 L:627 M:453 T:290
160. Patients with afibrinogenemia usually present with an abnormal: A. Bleeding time only. B. Reptilase time only. C. Thrombin time only. D. Bleeding time, reptilase time, and thrombin time.	D H:474 L:633 M:450 T:x

Select the Best Answer	Answers & References

161. The most sensitive test for heparin therapy and DIC is the:
    A. PT.
    B. APTT.
    C. Thrombin time.
    D. Bleeding time.
	C
	H:481
	L:614
	M:411
	T:396–397

162. Fever, thrombocytopenia, central nervous system damage, and renal disease are characteristic of:
    A. Primary fibrinolysis.
    B. Secondary fibrinolysis.
    C. Thrombotic thrombocytopenic purpura.
    D. Infectious liver disease.
	C
	H:495
	L:682
	M:226
	T:274

163. Heparin:
    A. Blocks the final synthesis step of vitamin K–dependent proteins.
    B. Reduces the circulating level of factor X.
    C. Binds with AT III to inhibit thrombin.
    D. Is removed from the blood via the liver.
	C
	H:510
	L:593
	M:401
	T:284

164. The vitamin K–dependent factors are:
    A. I, II, V, and VIII.
    B. II, V, VII, and X.
    C. II, VII, IX, and X.
    D. V, VII, VIII, and X.
	C
	H:432
	L:583
	M:386
	T:278

165. Factor deficiencies that individually may cause an elevated PT and APTT include:
    A. II, V, and VIII.
    B. II, V, and X.
    C. V, VII, and X.
    D. VII, VIII, and X.
	B
	H:432
	L:613
	M:450
	T:283

166. A patient whose abnormal PT is *not* corrected with either aged serum or adsorbed plasma reagent has a deficiency of factor:
    A. II.
    B. V.
    C. VII.
    D. X.
	A
	H:432
	L:613
	M:412
	T:x

167. A patient has a normal PT and an abnormal APTT, which is corrected with adsorbed plasma reagent but *not* aged serum. The patient has a deficiency of factor:
    A. VIII.
    B. IX.
    C. XI.
    D. XII.
	A
	H:432
	L:613
	M:412
	T:392

Select the Best Answer	Answers & References
168. A qualitative platelet defect will affect the: A. PT. B. APTT. C. Bleeding time. D. Platelet count.	C H:436 L:673 M:432 T:275
169. Which of the following factors is *not* found in aged serum? A. VII B. VIII C. IX D. X	B H:433 L:613 M:410 T:278
170. A diagnosis of essential thrombocythemia may be made once the platelet count exceeds _____ $\times 10^9$/L. A. 400 B. 500 C. 750 D. 1000	D H:446 L:440 M:297 T:x
171. Organs that sequester or destroy platelets include the: A. Spleen. B. Kidney. C. Liver and kidney. D. Endothelium system.	A H:449 L:663 M:429 T:271
172. A 62-year-old black male presents with schizocytes (schistocytes), thrombocytopenia, acute renal failure, and enlarged kidneys. The most likely diagnosis is: A. DIC. B. Thrombotic thrombocytopenic purpura. C. Hemolytic uremic syndrome. D. Acute renal failure.	C H:450 L:682 M:224 T:x
173. A patient with a bleeding diathesis shows an elevated APTT, decreased factor VIII assay, normal platelet aggregation with ADP, epinephrine, and thrombin, but reduced aggregation with ristocetin. The likely diagnosis is: A. Hemophilia A. B. Hemophilia B. C. Bernard-Soulier syndrome. D. von Willebrand's disease.	D H:470 L:630 M:443 T:289–290
174. A prolonged bleeding time is seen usually in which of the following? A. Afibrinogenemia B. Dysfibrinogenemia C. Hypofibrinogenemia D. Hyperfibrinogenemia	A H:474 L:673 M:450 T:x

Select the Best Answer	Answers & References

175. An elevated PT, APTT, and thrombin time in a patient with DIC is caused by:
   A. Circulating inhibitors.
   B. Hypofibrinogenemia and modification of factors V and VIII.
   C. An inability to utilize calcium.
   D. Consumption of factors X, XII, and XIII.
	B
	H:493
	L:x
	M:456
	T:283, 291

176. An autosomal dominant inheritance, easy bruising, and a prolonged bleeding time are consistent with:
   A. Glanzmann's thrombasthenia.
   B. DIC.
   C. von Willebrand's disease.
   D. Hemophilia A.
	C
	H:441
	L:630
	M:439, 442–443
	T:287

177. The myeloproliferative disorders include all the following *except*:
   A. Polycythemia vera.
   B. Chronic myelocytic leukemia.
   C. Glanzmann's thrombasthenia.
   D. Essential thrombocythemia.
	C
	H:446
	L:431
	M:277
	T:222

178. Several hours after birth, an infant develops petechiae purpuric hemorrhages, and a platelet count of 21×10^9/L. The most likely diagnosis is:
   A. Drug-induced immune thrombocytopenia.
   B. Secondary immune thrombocytopenia.
   C. Isoimmune neonatal thrombocytopenia.
   D. Neonatal idiopathic thrombocytopenic purpura.
	C
	H:454
	L:683
	M:x
	T:274

179. The average diameter of a normal platelet is _____ μm.
   A. 2–4
   B. 6–8
   C. 10–12
   D. 15–20
	A
	H:417
	L:660
	M:366
	T:269

180. The contact group of coagulation factors includes factors:
   A. X and XI.
   B. XI, XII, and prekallikrein.
   C. XII, XIII, and prekallikrein.
   D. XI, XII, and XIII.
	B
	H:426
	L:583
	M:386
	T:279

181. Thrombin enhances coagulation by:
   A. Converting fibrinogen to fibrin.
   B. Enhancing factor VII.
   C. Activating factor XII.
   D. Increasing thrombopoiesis.
	A
	H:428
	L:590
	M:398
	T:279

Select the Best Answer	Answers & References

182. Christmas factor is the synonym for factor:
  A. IX.
  B. X.
  C. XI.
  D. XII.
	A
	H:432
	L:582
	M:446
	T:278

183. The kinin system is involved in all the following *except*:
  A. Inflammation.
  B. Thrombopoiesis.
  C. Vascular permeability.
  D. Chemotaxis.
	B
	H:434
	L:582
	M:57
	T:x

184. Plasmin inhibitors:
  A. Interfere with in vitro coagulation tests.
  B. Prevent in vivo consumption of fibrinogen.
  C. Inactivate factors V and VIII.
  D. Disperse the fibrin monomer.
	B
	H:489
	L:x
	M:413
	T:282

185. Ingestion of aspirin will adversely affect the:
  A. Bleeding time.
  B. Platelet count.
  C. Prothrombin time.
  D. Activated partial thromboplastin time.
	A
	H:588
	L:673
	M:378
	T:388

186. Following aspirin ingestion, coagulation tests should be postponed for:
  A. 24 hours.
  B. 2–3 days.
  C. 1 week.
  D. 1 month.
	C
	H:588
	L:673
	M:437
	T:x

187. A patient with a congenital deficiency of antithrombin III, protein C, or protein S may exhibit:
  A. Superficial bruising.
  B. Venous thrombosis.
  C. Disseminated intravascular coagulation.
  D. Gingival bleeding.
	B
	H:504
	L:640–641
	M:465
	T:285–286

Select the Best Answer	Answers & References

188. A 45-year-old black male presents with the following lab results.

Laboratory Test	Normal Range	Patient
RBC count ($\times 10^{12}$/L)	4.5–6.0	6.8
Hemoglobin (g/L)	135–180	205
Hematocrit (L/L)	0.40–0.54	0.62

The patient's physician orders a PT and APTT. When the specimen is collected, how much of the patient's whole blood should be added to 0.5 mL of sodium citrate?

A. 3.4
B. 4.5
C. 7.1
D. 9.0

C
H:350
L:x
M:407
T:384

189. Platelet clumps and satellitism are seen on a smear from blood collected in EDTA. The best course of action is to:

A. Repeat the platelet count using sodium citrated blood.
B. Repeat the platelet count using heparinized blood.
C. Report the clumps and satellitism as significant.
D. Report the clumps as significant and do not report the satellitism.

A
H:529
L:509
M:432
T:x

190. Interpret the following laboratory data.

Laboratory Test	Normal Range	Patient
Patient data		23-year-old female who delivered a healthy newborn 1 hour ago develops postoperative bleeding
WBC ($\times 10^9$/L)	4.5–11.0	18.0
Hemoglobin (g/L)	120–160	95
Platelet count ($\times 10^9$/L)	140–415	52
Prothrombin time (s)	10.0–14.0	16.1
Activated partial thromboplastin time (s)	22–40	57
Thrombin time (s)	8–15	26
Fibrinogen (mg/dL)	155–405	112
Euglobulin lysis time (min)	No lysis in 120 min	95
D-Dimer (μg/mL)	<0.5	>2.0
Bleeding time (min)	2–9	12.5
Factor VIII assay (%)	50–150	112
Peripheral blood smear	Normocytic, normochromic	Schizocytes (schistocytes)

Select the Best Answer	Answers & References
The most likely diagnosis is: A. von Willebrand's disease. B. Circulating inhibitors. C. Normal postoperative phenomenon. D. Disseminated intravascular coagulation.	D H:585–612 L:635 M:457 T:292
191. A 71-year-old black female presents with a history of taking an oral anticoagulant for the past several months. Her prothrombin time is 63 s. Which of the following treatments would allow for the quickest correction of the prothrombin time? A. Vitamin K injections B. Protamine sulfate injections C. Fresh frozen plasma transfusions D. Discontinuing the oral anticoagulant	C H:475 L:650 M:470 T:x
192. A patient's WBC count is 13.6×10^9/L. The differential reveals 75 nucleated RBCs per 100 WBCs. The corrected WBC count is _____ $\times 10^9$/L. A. 1.8 B. 4.9 C. 7.8 D. 18.1	C H:547 L:328 M:x T:347
193. A male with sickle cell anemia had a RBC count of 2.55×10^{12}/L, hematocrit of 0.25 L/L, and 91 reticulocytes per 1000 RBCs. The corrected reticulocyte count is: A. 1.5%. B. 2.5%. C. 5.1%. D. 9.1%.	C H:530 L:116 M:89 T:61
194. Blood is pipetted to the 0.5 mark of a RBC pipet. The number of cells counted in the standard RBC squares of one side of a Neubauer hemacytometer is 198. The total RBC count is _____ $\times 10^{12}$/L. A. 0.90 B. 1.98 C. 3.96 D. 5.94	B H:526 L:318–322 M:x T:339–341
195. Blood is pipetted to the 1.0 mark of a WBC pipet. The number of cells counted in the standard WBC squares of one side of a Neubauer hemacytometer is 225. The total WBC count is _____ $\times 10^9$/L. A. 5.6 B. 11.3 C. 56.3 D. 112.5	A H:528 L:322 M:x T:345–347

Select the Best Answer	Answers & References

196. A complete blood count on a patient reveals the following data.
 	
   WBC $(\times 10^9/L) = 26$
   Differential:
 	
   Segmented neutrophils   63%
   Band neutrophils   11%
   Lymphocytes   15%
   Monocytes   7%
   Eosinophils   4%
 	
 The absolute neutrophil count is _____ $\times 10^9/L$.
 	
   A. 16.4
   B. 19.2
   C. 20.3
   D. 22.1
	B
	H:530
	L:328
	M:52
	T:137

197. The following is a 500-cell bone marrow differential.
 	
   Myeloblasts   8
   Promyelocytes   13
   Myelocytes   99
   Metamyelocytes   65
   Segmented neutrophils   97
   Rubriblasts   3
   Prorubricytes   18
   Rubricytes   91
   Metarubricytes   29
   Lymphocytes   63
   Plasma cells   3
   Monocytes   11
 	
 The M : E ratio is:
 	
   A. 1 : 2
   B. 2 : 1
   C. 1 : 2.5
   D. 2.5 : 1
	B
	H:49–50
	L:377
	M:101
	T:356

For questions: 198–200:
 	
 WBC $= 14.7 \times 10^9/L$
 RBC $= 3.81 \times 10^{12}/L$
 Hb $= 113$ g/L
 Hct $= 0.359$ L/L
 	
 198. The MCV is _____ fL.
 	
   A. 9.4
   B. 28.9
   C. 31.5
   D. 94.2
	D
	H:532
	L:113
	M:86
	T:76

Select the Best Answer	Answers & References

199. The MCH is ____ pg.
    A. 22.1
    B. 29.7
    C. 31.5
    D. 76.9
	B
	H:532
	L:114
	M:87
	T:76

200. The MCHC is ____ g/L.
    A. 221
    B. 297
    C. 315
    D. 769
	C
	H:532
	L:114
	M:87
	T:76

Refer to the color plates for the following questions.	

201. Color Plate 1. If this cell morphology was observed, the next step would be to:
    A. Have the blood recollected.
    B. Remake the peripheral blood smear.
    C. Perform a sickle solubility test.
    D. Perform an erythrocyte sedimentation test.
	C
	H:150
	L:198
	M:141
	T:111

202. Color Plate 2. If this cell morphology was observed, the next step would be to perform a(n):
    A. Hemoglobin electrophoresis.
    B. Kleihauer-Betke stain.
    C. Iron stain.
    D. Heat denaturation test.
	A
	H:151
	L:198
	M:140
	T:111

203. Color Plate 3. What is the best description of the WBC?
    A. Variant lymphocyte
    B. Toxic granulation
    C. Pyknotic nucleus
    D. Hypersegmentation
	D
	H:Plate 66
	L:341
	M:169
	T:Plate 40

204. Color Plate 4. What disorder could the WBC morphology indicate?
    A. Infectious mononucleosis
    B. Acute myelocytic leukemia
    C. Bacterial infection
    D. Multiple myeloma
	A
	H:Plate 136
	L:352
	M:269
	T:158

205. Color Plate 5. Identify the WBC indicated by the arrow.
    A. Variant lymphocyte
    B. Monocyte
    C. Lymphoblast
    D. Metamyelocyte
	B
	H:Plate 31
	L:Plate 10
	M:Plate II-N
	T:Plate 35

Select the Best Answer	Answers & References

206. Color Plate 6. An elevation of the pictured WBCs may indicate:
    A. Viral infection.
    B. Parasitic infestation.
    C. Pelger-Huët anomaly.
    D. May-Hegglin anomaly.
	C
	H:Plate 132
	L:357
	M:259
	T:Plate 41

207. Color Plate 7. What is the disorder suggested by the WBC morphology?
    A. Acute lymphocytic leukemia
    B. Chronic lymphocytic leukemia
    C. Acute myelocytic leukemia
    D. Chronic myelocytic leukemia
	B
	H:Plate 180
	L:456
	M:359
	T:Plate 51

208. Color Plate 8. What is the disorder suggested by the WBC morphology?
    A. Acute lymphocytic leukemia
    B. Chronic lymphocytic leukemia
    C. Acute myelocytic leukemia
    D. Chronic myelocytic leukemia
	C
	H:Plate 140, 149
	L:Plate 42
	M:Plate IV-A
	T:Plates 54, 59

209. Color Plate 9. Identify cell A.
    A. Large platelet
    B. Lymphocyte
    C. Monocyte
    D. Blast
	A
	H:358
	L:Plate 53
	M:368
	T:Plate 76

210. Color Plate 9. Identify cell B.
    A. Platelet
    B. Metamyelocyte
    C. Lymphocyte
    D. Nucleated RBC
	D
	H:Plate 9
	L:Plate 3
	M:Plate I-D
	T:Plate 5

211. Color Plate 10. Identify the nucleated cells.
    A. Metamyelocytes
    B. Variant lymphocytes
    C. Prorubricytes
    D. Blasts
	B
	H:Plate 136
	L:Plate 26
	M:Plate III-A
	T:Plate 49

212. Color Plate 11. What is the best morphologic description?
    A. Thrombocytosis
    B. Platelet agglutination
    C. Platelet satellitism
    D. Megakaryocytosis
	C
	H:529
	L:28, 30
	M:432
	T:x

Select the Best Answer	Answers & References

213. Color Plate 12. What is the predominant RBC morphology?
   A. Codocytes (target cells)
   B. Discocytes (normal RBCs)
   C. Schizocytes (schistocytes)
   D. Stomatocytes
	A
	H:Plate 126
	L:94
	M:93
	T:Plate 16

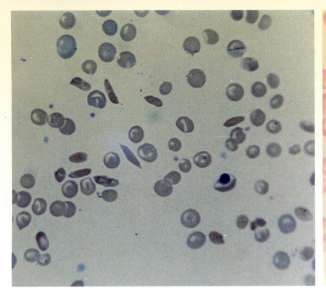

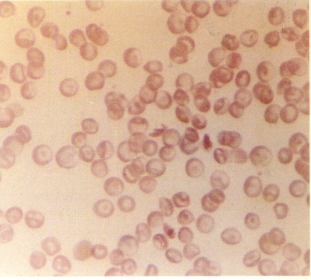

Color Plate 1   Color Plate 2

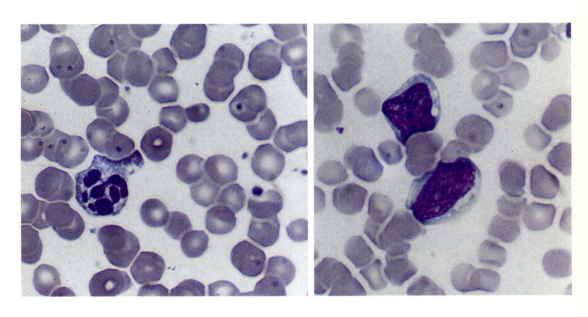

Color Plate 3   Color Plate 4

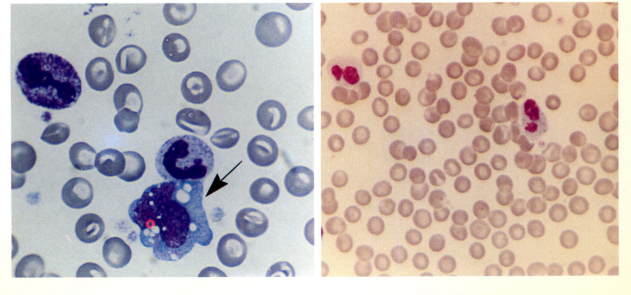

Color Plate 5   Color Plate 6

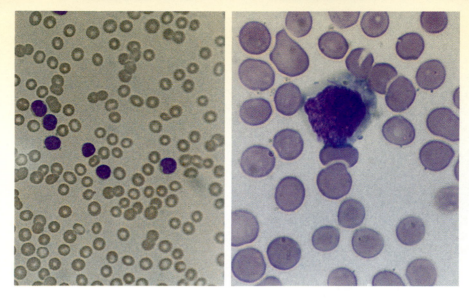

Color Plate 7

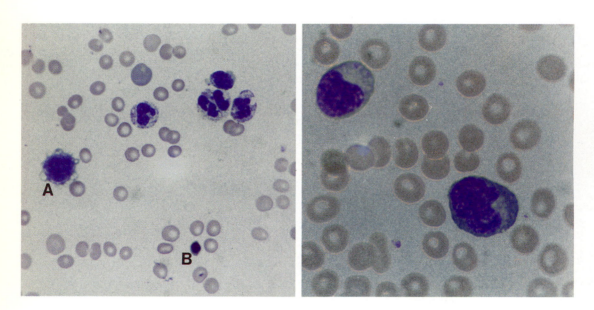

Color Plate 8

Color Plate 9

Color Plate 10

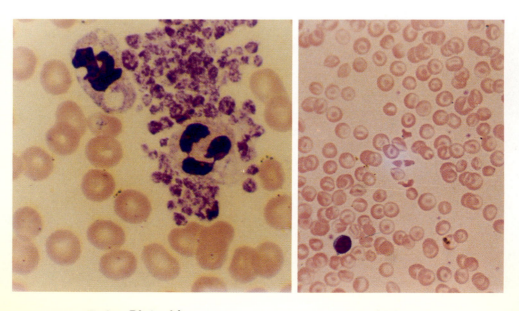

Color Plate 11

Color Plate 12

Appendix D

Glossary

Abetalipoproteinemia: Autosomal recessive disorder in which a beta-lipoprotein deficiency results in RBC membrane abnormalities and other systemic abnormalities

Acanthocyte: RBC with a few irregular spines protruding from the cell surface

Achlorhydria: Reduced hydrochloric acid in gastric secretions; often associated with pernicious anemia

Acidified serum lysis (Ham's) test: Measure of complement sensitivity of RBCs; often associated with paroxysmal nocturnal hemoglobinuria

Activated partial thromboplastin time: Screening test for abnormalities in the intrinsic coagulation pathway and for monitoring heparin therapy

Activated whole blood clotting time: Screening test for abnormalities in the intrinsic coagulation pathway

Acute: Disorder with rapid onset and progression

Adhesion: First step in platelet plug formation; platelets cohering to surfaces other than platelets

ADPase: Enzyme produced by endothelial cells and capable of degrading ADP

Adsorbed plasma: Plasma that has been treated with aluminum hydroxide or barium sulfate; the resulting plasma contains coagulation factors I, V, VIII, XI, XII, and XIII

Afibrinogenemia: Hereditary or acquired absence of fibrinogen (factor I)

Aged serum: Serum that has been stored; factors that are consumed during clotting or are labile are not present; aged serum contains coagulation factors VII, IX, X, XI, and XII

Agglutination: Disorderly clumps of cells or particles

Agglutinin: See antibody

Agglutinogen: See antigen

Aggregation: Platelets cohering to other platelets

AIDS: Acquired immunodeficiency syndrome

Alder-Reilly anomaly: Autosomal recessive disorder that prevents the normal breakdown of mucopolysaccharides; the undegraded substance is deposited as non-transient, dark-staining granules in the cytoplasm of neutrophils and monocytes

Alpha-1-antitrypsin: Naturally occurring plasma protein that acts as an anticoagulant by inhibiting serine proteases

Alpha-2-antiplasmin: Naturally occurring inhibitor of fibrinolysis

Alpha-2-macroglobulin: Naturally occurring protein that inhibits plasmin, thrombin, and kallikrein, as well as other serine proteases

Alpha granules: Platelet organelles containing substances necessary for hemostasis

Androgens: Endocrine secretions that produce male characteristics

Anemia: Less than normal numbers of RBCs

Anisocytosis: Variation in RBC size; the RDW usually exceeds 14.5 percent

Antibody: Protein produced in response to antigen stimulation

Anticoagulant: Natural or acquired substance that inhibits blood clotting

Antigen: Any substance capable of eliciting an immune response and reacting with the products of that response

Antihemophilic factor A: Coagulation factor VIII; cofactor in the coagulation mechanism

Antihemophilic factor B: Coagulation factor IX; inactive precursor to a serine protease which aids in the conversion of factor X to the active state

Antihuman globulin test: See indirect antihuman globulin test and direct antihuman globulin test

Antiplatelet antibodies: Antibodies against platelet antigens

Antithrombin III: Coagulation inhibitor of thrombin and factors IXa, Xa, and XIa

Aplasia: Aberrant or deficient development of cells within an organ such as blood cells within the bone marrow

APTT: Activated partial thromboplastin time

Artery: Thick-walled, resilient vessel in which oxygenated blood flows away from the heart to the tissues

Aspirin tolerance test: Measure of prolongation of the bleeding time following aspirin ingestion; the test is often excessively prolonged in von Willebrand's disease

Asynchrony: Maturation rates of a cell's nucleus and cytoplasm differ

Auer bodies: Aggregates of primary granules seen in myeloblasts and monoblasts of acute leukemia

Autoagglutinin: Antibody produced to the person's own antigens and causing clumping of affected cells

Babesia: Parasitic protozoan that infects RBCs

Band neutrophil: Fifth in the maturation sequence of the granulocyte; it is distinguished from the earlier cell by the horseshoe- or sausage-shaped nucleus

Basophil: Mature granulocytic WBC with a segmented nucleus and coarse, dark-staining, cytoplasmic granules

Basophilia: Absolute basophil count above 0.3×10^9/liter

Basophilic normoblast: See prorubricyte

Basophilic stippling: Coarse granulation in the RBC caused by RNA aggregates

Bence-Jones protein: Heat-sensitive protein found in the urine of multiple myeloma patients; the protein precipitates when heated to 45 to 55°C, redissolves at 100°C, then reappears when cooled

Bernard-Soulier syndrome: Inherited platelet disorder in which adhesion is abnormal

Bilirubin: Bile pigment produced during heme degradation

Blast: Earliest recognizable cell of any cell line

Bleeding time: Measure of capillary fragility and platelet function

Blister cell: RBC with a vacuole, resembling a blister, near the membrane surface

B lymphocyte: WBC differentiated by the bone marrow and responsible for humoral immunity

Buffy coat: Layer of WBCs and platelets at the RBC-plasma interface after whole blood is centrifuged

Burr cell: RBC with irregular spiny projections on the surface of the cell

C1 inactivator: Naturally occurring anticoagulant that inhibits plasmin and C1 esterase in the complement pathway

Cabot ring: RBC inclusion appearing as thread-like round, oval, or figure-eight loops; the rings are thought to be remnants of nuclear membrane

Capillary: Thin-walled vessel that carries blood from small arteries to small veins

Carboxyhemoglobin: Hemoglobin molecule carrying carbon monoxide

CBC: Complete blood count

Cellularity: Number of hematopoietic cells; estimated by comparing the fat cell to nucleated hematopoietic cell ratio

Chédiak-Higashi syndrome: Autosomal recessive disorder resulting in large acidophilic lysosomes in the cytoplasm of WBCs, in addition to systemic problems leading to death

Chemotactic factors: Substances that attract phagocytic cells to the site of infection or injury

Christmas factor: Coagulation factor IX

Chromatin: Network of DNA and basic proteins of the nucleus

Chronic: Disorder with an insidious onset and slow progression

Circulating pool: WBCs moving freely in the peripheral blood

Clot retraction: Measure of platelet quantity and function

Codocyte: Target cell; RBC that shows hemoglobin concentrations at the outer rim and center of the cell; a pale circular zone separates the two areas

Cofactor: Component that aids in conversion of a zymogen to the active enzyme

Collagen: Structural protein produced by the endothelium and capable of activating coagulation factors and stimulating platelet adhesion

Colony-stimulating factors: Substances that promote the proliferation and differentiation of stem cells

Common pathway: Part of the coagulation mechanism that may be activated by either the intrinsic or extrinsic pathways; it includes factors X, V, II, and I

Complement: System of proteins that mediate immune cytolysis as well as participate in other functions

Contact family: Coagulation factors XI, XII, prekallikrein, and high-molecular-weight kininogen

Coumarin drugs: Derivatives include coumarin, dicoumerol, and warfarin; anticoagulants that interfere with the synthesis of the prothrombin family by competing for vitamin K; therapy is monitored with prothrombin times

Cryoglobulin: Proteins that precipitate at low temperatures and redissolve when warmed to body temperature

Cyanmethemoglobin: Stable compound produced during the spectrophotometric assay of hemoglobin

Dacryocyte: Teardrop cell; elongated RBC rounded on one end and pointed on the other end

D-Dimer: Cross-linked fragment of fibrin monomers resulting from fibrin degradation

Dense bodies: Platelet organelles containing substances necessary for hemostasis

Deoxyhemoglobin: Hemoglobin molecule with iron in the ferrous (Fe^{2+}) state and not carrying oxygen

Diapedesis: Movement of cells through intact vessel walls into tissues

DIC: Disseminated intravascular coagulation

Differential: Categorization of the types of nucleated cells present in bone marrow, peripheral blood, or body fluid

Diffusely basophilic erythrocyte: See reticulocyte

2,3-Diphosphoglycerate (2,3-DPG): Molecule that enhances the release of oxygen from hemoglobin to tissues

Direct antiglobulin test: Measure of in vivo attachment of antibodies to RBC antigens

Discocyte: Normal RBC; bi-concave disc with no nucleus

Disseminated intravascular coagulation: Bleeding disorder secondary to widespread clotting in the peripheral circulation; numerous clots consume coagulation factors and platelets, as well as initiate fibrinolysis; uncontrolled bleeding ensues

Döhle body: Pale-blue–staining areas within the cytoplasm of mature neutrophils and consisting of RNA; often associated with bacterial infections

Donath-Landsteiner antibody: Bi-thermal antibody, anti-P, which is often produced following a viral infection and causes paroxysmal cold hemoglobinuria

Drepanocyte: Sickle cell; elongated RBC with pointed projections on both ends

Dysfibrinogenemia: Congenital disorder producing abnormal fibrinogen molecules

EACA: Epsilon aminocaproic acid

Ecchymoses: Large venous hemorrhages into subcutaneous tissue

Echinocyte: RBC with regularly spaced bumps protruding from the cell surface

EDTA: See Ethylenediaminetetraacetic acid

Ehlers-Danlos syndrome: Congenital disorder of platelet adhesion created by abnormal collagen

Elliptocyte: Ovalocyte; RBC with bi-polar aggregates of hemoglobin which cause the cell to be slightly to severely elongated

Embden-Meyerhof glycolytic pathway: Anaerobic metabolic pathway providing 90 percent of the RBC's energy requirement

Embolus: Clot carried by blood circulation to a small vessel resulting in vessel obstruction

Endomitosis: Nuclear division without cellular division

Endothelium: Innermost layer of blood vessels

Eosinopenia: Absolute eosinophil count below 0.05×10^9/liter

Eosinophil: Mature granulocyte with a segmented nucleus and large orange-staining granules

Eosinophilia: Absolute eosinophil count above 0.7×10^9/liter

Epistaxis: Nosebleed

Epsilon aminocaproic acid (EACA): Therapeutic agent used to inhibit plasminogen activators

Erythrocyte: Cell capable of carrying oxygen to tissues; also known as red blood cell

Erythrocyte sedimentation rate (ESR): Measurement of the RBC settling rate in a column of whole blood

Erythropoiesis: Production of RBCs

Erythropoietin: Substance of renal origin that stimulates production of RBCs

ESR: Erythrocyte sedimentation rate

Ethylenediaminetetraacetic acid (EDTA): Anticoagulant commonly used for collection of hematology specimens. It acts as a calcium chelator, thus deleting a vital component of the coagulation mechanism.

Euglobulin lysis time: Measure of clot integrity

Extramedullary hematopoiesis: Production of blood cells outside of the bone marrow cavities

Extravascular hemolysis: RBC destruction occurring outside the blood vessels

Extrinsic coagulation pathway: Coagulation mechanisms initiated by contact between tissue thromboplastin (factor III) and factor VII; it also includes factors X, V, II, and I

FAB: French-American-British classification system for leukemias

Factor assay: Quantitative measurement of a specific coagulation factor

Fanconi's anemia: Congenital disorder producing bone marrow hypoplasia which is evident as pancytopenia in the circulating blood; other physical abnormalities also are seen

Ferritin: Storage form of iron

Fibrin: Insoluble protein that occurs when thrombin acts on fibrinogen

Fibrin stabilizing factor: Coagulation factor XIII; inactive precursor to a transaminase that stabilizes polymerized fibrin monomers in the initial clot

Fibrinogen: Substrate in the coagulation mechanism that is converted to fibrin

Fibrinogen family: Coagulation factors I, V, VIII, and XIII

Fibrin(ogen) split products: By-products that occur when fibrinogen or fibrin is degraded by plasmin

Fibrinolysis: Fibrin degradation by enzymes

Fibrinopeptides: Fragments split from fibrinogen

Fitzgerald factor: See high-molecular-weight kininogen

Flame cell: Plasma cell with pinkish-red cytoplasm

Fletcher factor: See prekallikrein

Gaucher's disease: Autosomal recessive disorder causing a deficiency of beta-glucocerebrosidase, which is necessary for lipid metabolism; failure to break down lipids results in large macrophages with wrinkled-looking cytoplasm and small, off-centered nuclei

Glanzmann's thrombasthenia: Inherited deficiency of a platelet glycoprotein resulting in abnormal platelet aggregation

Globin: Amino acid chains in hemoglobin

Glossitis: Inflammation of the tongue

Glucose-6-phosphate dehydrogenase (G6PD): Enzyme in the hexose monophosphate shunt that is ultimately responsible for reducing hydrogen peroxide to water in cells; failure of this mechanism results in denatured hemoglobin and hemolytic anemia

Glycocalyx: Substance produced by the endothelium; it coats the endothelial cells with heparan sulfate to help prevent thrombosis

G6PD: Glucose-6-phosphate dehydrogenase

Granulocytes: Cells that mature into neutrophils, eosinophils, or basophils

Hageman factor: Coagulation factor XII; inactive precursor to a serine protease in the intrinsic coagulation pathway

Ham's test: See acidified serum lysis test

Haptoglobin: Glycoprotein required for clearance of free hemoglobin from the body

Heinz body: RBC cytoplasmic inclusion appearing as dark-staining, round areas. The inclusion is the result of denatured hemoglobin and is seen only with supravital stains

Helmet cell: Fragmented RBC that appears to have a piece of the cell removed; thus, it resembles a helmet

Hemacytometer: Chamber used for manually counting cells

Hemarthrosis: Bleeding into a joint cavity

Hematocrit: Measure of the volume of packed RBCs to total volume of blood

Hematology: Study of the concentration and morphology of blood cells and their precursors

Hematoma: Blood that has escaped from vessels into a localized area of tissue. The blood is usually clotted.

Hematopoiesis: Production and maturation of blood cells

Heme: Component of hemoglobin containing porphyrin rings and iron

Hemoglobin: Protein usually confined to the RBC and capable of carrying oxygen in the blood

Hemoglobin A: Hemoglobin containing two alpha and two beta globin chains

Hemoglobin Bart's: Hemoglobin containing four gamma globin chains instead of two alpha and two beta chains

Hemoglobin C: Hemoglobin containing a defective beta globin chain in which lysine is substituted for glutamic acid at the sixth amino acid position

Hemoglobin C crystal: Oblong hexagonal crystal that distorts the RBC membrane; it is the result of an abnormal beta globin chain in hemoglobin

Hemoglobin D: Hemoglobin containing a defective beta globin chain in which glycine is substituted for glutamic acid at the one hundred twenty-first amino acid position

Hemoglobin E: Hemoglobin containing a defective beta globin chain in which lysine is substituted for glutamic acid at the twenty-sixth amino acid position

Hemoglobin F: Hemoglobin containing two alpha and two gamma globin chains

Hemoglobin H: Hemoglobin containing four beta globin chains instead of two alpha and two beta chains

Hemoglobin M: Hemoglobin in which an amino acid substitution in the globin chain causes the hemoglobin iron to remain in the ferric (Fe^{3+}) form instead of the ferrous (Fe^{2+}) form

Hemoglobin S: Hemoglobin containing a defective beta globin chain in which valine is substituted for glutamic acid at the sixth amino acid position

Hemoglobinemia: Hemoglobin released into the plasma

Hemoglobinopathy: Disorder in which the hemoglobin has an abnormal structure or is produced in abnormal quantities

Hemolysis: RBC destruction

Hemolytic disease of the newborn: Destruction of fetal RBCs caused by attachment of maternal antibodies to fetal RBC antigens

Hemopexin: Serum protein that binds heme

Hemophilia: Hereditary disorder marked by bleeding episodes

Hemorrhage: Blood loss due to a ruptured vessel

Hemorrhagic disease of the newborn: Bleeding episodes in the newborn due to inadequate vitamin K availability leading to a deficiency of vitamin K–dependent coagulation factors

Hemosiderin: Water-insoluble storage iron

Hemostasis: Cessation of bleeding

Heparin: Anticoagulant that enhances the action of antithrombin III; therapy is monitored with the activated partial thromboplastin time.

Heparin-associated thrombocytopenia: Reduced platelet count during heparin therapy

Hepatomegaly: Enlargement of the liver

Hepatosplenomegaly: Enlargement of the liver and spleen

Hereditary hemorrhagic telangiectasia: Deficiency of vessel elastic fibers that results in abnormal capillary dilation

Hereditary persistence of fetal hemoglobin: Congenital disorder in which the "switchover" from gamma globin chains to beta globin chains fails

Hexosaminidase A: Enzyme that may be deficient in patients with Tay-Sachs disease

Hexose monophosphate shunt: Aerobic metabolic pathway providing 10 percent of the RBC's energy requirement; also known as the pentose phosphate pathway

High-molecular-weight kininogen: Cofactor involved in contact activation of the intrinsic coagulation pathway

HIV: Human immunodeficiency virus

Hodgkin's disease: Malignant lymphoma characterized by Reed-Sternberg cells in lymph nodes

Howell-Jolly body: RBC inclusion appearing as eccentric, small, round, non-refractile, purple masses and consisting of DNA

Hydrocytosis: Hereditary RBC defect that allows water to enter the RBC; the RBC will appear as a stomatocyte

Hyperplasia: Increased growth of cells within tissue

Hypersegmentation: Segmented neutrophils with more than five lobes

Hypochromasia: RBC with greater than one third central pallor; the MCHC is usually less than 32 grams per liter

Hypogammaglobulinemia: Decreased production of gamma globulins

Hypoplasia: Decreased growth of cells within tissue

Hypoxia: Oxygen deficiency

Icterus: Jaundice; yellow pigmentation of skin, mucosa, and body excretions due to elevated bilirubin levels

Immune thrombocytopenic purpura: Acquired disorder in which antibodies are produced against platelet antigens

Immunoglobulin: See antibody

Indirect antiglobulin test: Measure of the in vitro attachment of antibodies to RBC antigens

Insidious: Appearing or changing gradually

Interleukin: Protein necessary for lymphocyte production

International normalized ratio: Method for reporting prothrombin time. It is calculated by the following formula: $[\text{Patient time} \div \text{reference time mean}]^{\text{ISI}}$, where ISI is the International Sensitivity Index supplied by the reagent manufacturer.

Intravascular hemolysis: RBC destruction occurring inside the blood vessels

Intrinsic coagulation pathway: Coagulation mechanism that begins with contact activation of factor XII and includes factors XI, IX, VIII, X, V, II, and I

Intrinsic factor: Glycoprotein secreted by parietal cells of the stomach and necessary for vitamin B_{12} absorption

Isoimmune: Possessing an antibody against an antigen within the same system

Karyorrhexis: Ruptured, cloverleaf-shaped nucleus indicating cellular degeneration

Karyotype: Procedure used to arrange mitotic chromosomes in descending order of size; abnormalities then can be evaluated

Keloid: Excessive scar formation

Keratocyte: RBC with extreme shape change including variable numbers of spines and spurs projecting from the membrane

Kleihauer-Betke stain: Special stain that uses acid elution to denature all hemoglobins in the RBC except fetal hemoglobin; the presence and distribution of fetal hemoglobin can be evaluated

Knizocyte: Triangle cell; RBC that looks pinched into a triangular shape

LE cell: Neutrophil that has engulfed a nucleus that has been degraded by antinuclear antibody; associated with lupus erythematosus

Lee-White whole blood clotting time: Screening test for abnormalities in the intrinsic coagulation pathway

Left shift: See shift to the left

Leptocyte: RBC that resembles a codocyte but is thinner, yielding a small rim of hemoglobin at the edge of the cell

Leukemia: Malignant transformation of blood-forming cells; may be acute or chronic and may affect any hematopoietic cell line

Leukemoid reaction: Increased WBC count with immature cells; due to infections or inflammation; may be confused with leukemia

Leukocyte: White blood cell

Leukocyte alkaline phosphatase: Enzyme present in the normal, mature neutrophil but decreased in neutrophils of chronic myelocytic leukemia

Leukocytosis: Absolute WBC count above $10.8 \times 10^9/L$

Leukoerythroblastosis: Abnormal immature WBCs, RBCs, and platelets

Leukopenia: Absolute WBC count below $4.4 \times 10^9/L$

Leukopoiesis: Production of WBCs

Leukotreine: Compound involved in immediate hypersensitivity reactions

Lipemia: Increase in blood lipids

Luebering-Rapoport pathway: RBC pathway that produces 2,3-DPG

Lupus erythematosus: Connective tissue disorder producing antinuclear antibodies

Lymphadenopathy: Disorder of the lymph nodes

Lymphocyte: WBC responsible for cellular or humoral immunity; see B lymphocyte and T lymphocyte

Lymphocytosis: Absolute lymphocyte count above $4.5 \times 10^9/L$

Lymphoid stem cell: Earliest cell in the lymphocytic cell line

Lymphoma: Malignant disorder of lymphoid tissue

Lymphopenia: Absolute lymphocyte count below $1.2 \times 10^9/L$

Lymphoproliferative disorder: Abnormal production of lymphocytes or plasma cells

M0: Acute undifferentiated leukemia

M1: Acute myelomonocytic leukemia without maturation

M2: Acute myelocytic leukemia with maturation

M3: Acute promyelocytic leukemia

M4: Acute myelomonocytic leukemia

M5: Acute monocytic leukemia

M6: Erythroleukemia

M7: Acute megakaryocytic leukemia

Macrocyte: RBC that is larger than normal (>8 micrometers in diameter or >98 femtoliters in volume)

Macrophage: Large phagocytic cell developing from the monocyte

Malaria: *Plasmodium* infestation of RBCs

Marginating pool: WBCs lining the walls of blood vessels

Mast cell: Tissue basophil

May-Hegglin anomaly: Autosomal dominant disorder characterized by abnormal platelets, thrombocytopenia, and pale-blue, Döhle-like inclusions in neutrophils

MCH: Mean cell hemoglobin

MCHC: Mean cell hemoglobin concentration

MCV: Mean cell volume

Mean cell hemoglobin (MCH): Calculated average of the amount of hemoglobin in an RBC

Mean cell hemoglobin concentration (MCHC): Calculated average concentration of hemoglobin in a volume of packed RBCs

Mean cell volume (MCV): Calculated or directly measured average of the individual RBC volume

Medullary hematopoiesis: Blood cell production inside the bone marrow cavities

Megakaryoblast: Earliest recognizable cell in the thrombocytic series

Megakaryocyte: Large, multinucleated, platelet-producing cell in the bone marrow

Megaloblast: Large, abnormal NRBC with a webby chromatin pattern

Megaloblastic: Term describing large NRBCs with abnormal morphology associated with B_{12} or folate deficiency

Megaloblastoid: Changes in RBC morphology that resemble megaloblastic disease but usually are due to malignant transformation

Metamegakaryocyte: Mature cell in the thrombocytic series

Metamyelocyte: Intermediate cell in the maturation sequence of the granulocyte. It is distinguished from the earlier cell by the indented (kidney-shaped) nucleus and the absence of nucleoli.

Metarubricyte: Most mature nucleated RBC; the nucleus is extremely condensed and pyknotic; the cytoplasm is bluish-pink

Methemalbumin: Component formed following intravascular hemolysis and consisting of albumin bound to heme

Methemoglobin: Hemoglobin molecule in the ferric (Fe^{3+}) state and incapable of carrying oxygen

Methemoglobin reductase pathway: System in the RBC that maintains iron in the ferrous (Fe^{2+}) state

Microcyte: RBC that is smaller than normal (<6 micrometers in diameter or <80 femtoliters in volume)

Monoblast: Earliest recognizable cell in the monocytic series

Monoclonal gammopathy: Plasma cell disorder that produces a single class of antibody and shows a spike in one region on protein electrophoresis

Monocyte: Mature cell of the monocytic series; it is mononuclear and capable of phagocytosis

Monocytopenia: Absolute monocyte count below 0.2×10^9/L

Monocytosis: Absolute monocyte count above 0.9×10^9/L

Mott cell: Plasma cell containing multiple Russell bodies

Mucopolysaccharidoses: Group of related disorders in which mucopolysaccharides are not degraded; the degradation failure results in WBCs with Alder-Reilly granules, as well as multiple systemic abnormalities

Multiple myeloma: Monoclonal gammopathy resulting from a malignant neoplasm of plasma cells

Myeloblast: Earliest recognizable cell in the granulocytic series

Myelocyte: Intermediate cell in the maturation sequence of the granulocyte; it is distinguished from the earlier cell by the presence of secondary granules

Myelodysplastic: Abnormal production and maturation of granulocytic, megakaryocytic, monocytic, or erythrocytic cells

Myeloid:erythroid (M:E) ratio: Total number of granulocytes and their precursors in the bone marrow divided by the total number of NRBCs in the bone marrow

Myeloperoxidase: Enzyme useful in differentiating immature myelocytic and monocytic cells from immature lymphocytic cells

Myeloproliferative disease: Abnormal production of granulocytes, monocytes, RBCs, or platelets

Neutropenia: Absolute neutrophil count below 1.5×10^9/L
Neutrophil: Granulocytic WBC with neutral-staining granules
Neutrophilia: Absolute neutrophil count above 6.5×10^9/L
Niemann-Pick disease: Autosomal recessive disorder causing a deficiency of sphingomyelinase; the failure to break down lipids results in large macrophages with foamy looking cytoplasm
Normochromic: RBCs that are normal in color (have one third central pallor)
Normocytic: RBCs that are normal in size (6 to 8 micrometers)
NRBC: Nucleated red blood cells
Nucleolus: Nuclear structure that is the site of RNA synthesis

Oncogene: Gene that, upon activation, aids in transformation of normal cells to tumor cells
Ontogeny: Maturation and development of a cell
Opsonins: Antibodies that enhance phagocytosis
Organomegaly: Enlargement of an organ of the body
Orthochromatic normoblast: See metarubricyte
Osmotic fragility: Measure of RBC sensitivity to varying concentrations of saline
Osteoclast: Large cell with multiple nuclei often linked to bone resorption
Ovalocyte: See elliptocyte
Oxyhemoglobin: Hemoglobin molecule in the ferrous (Fe^{2+}) state and carrying oxygen

Pallor: Lack of color
Pancytopenia: Decrease in all blood cells
Pappenheimer bodies: See siderotic granules
Paroxysmal cold hemoglobinuria: Acquired hemolytic anemia resulting from attachment of anti-P to corresponding RBC antigens; production of the antibody usually is transient and follows a viral infection
Paroxysmal nocturnal hemoglobinuria: Acquired structural or biochemical defect in the RBC, granulocyte, and platelet membranes that causes the cells to be hypersensitive to complement fixation
PCH: Paroxysmal cold hemoglobinuria
Pelger-Huët anomaly: Acquired disorder or autosomal dominant syndrome that produces a predominance of bi-lobed or non-segmented granulocytes; the acquired disorder usually precedes a neoplastic transformation, but the inherited form is benign
Pentose phosphate shunt: See hexose monophosphate shunt
Pernicious anemia: Disorder in which intrinsic factor is missing; the deficiency results in insufficient uptake of vitamin B_{12} which, in turn, leads to megaloblastic anemia
Petechiae: Minute hemorrhages from small vessels
Phagocytosis: Act of ingesting and degrading particles
Philadelphia chromosome: Abnormally small chromosome 22 resulting from a translocation of genetic material from chromosome 22 to chromosome 9; often associated with chronic myelocytic leukemia
Pince-nez cell: Bi-lobed neutrophil that may be seen in the Pelger-Huët anomaly
Plasma cell: WBC derived from B lymphocytes, responsible for humoral immunity, and not usually found in circulating blood
Plasmacytoid lymphocyte: WBC with characteristics of both the lymphocyte and the plasma cell
Plasmacytosis: Increased production of plasma cells
Plasmapheresis: Removal of blood from a donor with subsequent return of the cellular elements and retention of the plasma
Plasma thromboplastin antecedent: Coagulation factor XI; inactive precursor to a serine protease in the intrinsic coagulation pathway
Plasmin: Serine protease that degrades coagulation factors I, V, VIII, and fibrin
Plasminogen: Inert glycoprotein that may be converted to plasmin by fibrinolytic activators
Plasmodium: See malaria
Platelet: Disc-shaped, cytoplasmic fragment of a megakaryocyte; aids in blood coagulation
Platelet factor 3: Platelet membrane phospholipid required for hemostasis
Platelet neutralization procedure: Tests for the presence of lupus anticoagulants
Platelet retention: Measure of the platelets' abilities to adhere to foreign surfaces
Plateletpheresis: Removal of platelets from a donor
Pluripotential: Capable of developing into one of several different cell lines
PNH: Paroxysmal nocturnal hemoglobinuria

Poikilocytosis: Variation in RBC shape

Polychromasia: RBCs with bluish-tinged cytoplasm indicative of residual RNA

Polychromatophilic normoblast: See rubricyte

Polyclonal gammopathy: Reactive plasmacytosis that produces more than one type of antibody; protein electrophoresis shows a broad band in the gamma region

Polycythemia: Increased number of RBCs in the blood

Polyploidy: More than one nucleus (set of homologous chromosomes) in a cell

Porphyria: Disorder of heme synthesis

Porphyrin crystal: RBC cytoplasmic inclusion appearing as a needle-like, bluish rod and consisting of non-heme porphyrin

Prekallikrein: Inactive precursor to a serine protease that connects the coagulation pathways to fibrinolysis and kininogen activation

Primary fibrinolysis: Hemostatic disorder caused by excess plasminogen activators

Proaccelerin: Coagulation factor V; inactive precursor to a cofactor that speeds the transformation of pro-thrombin to thrombin

Proconvertin: Coagulation factor VII; inactive precursor to an enzyme that activates factor X

Prolymphocyte: Intermediate precursor in the maturation sequence of the lymphocyte; the chromatin clumping renders nucleoli less visible than in the earlier stage

Promegakaryocyte: Intermediate precursor in the thrombocytic cell line; the cell size and nuclear number is increased over the cell of an earlier stage

Promonocyte: Intermediate precursor in the maturation sequence of the monocyte; the nucleus displays a foamy appearance and the cytoplasm is grayer than the earlier stage

Promyelocyte: Intermediate precursor in the maturation sequence of the granulocyte; it is distinguished from the earlier cell by the presence of primary granules

Pronormoblast: See rubriblast

Prorubricyte: Intermediate precursor in the maturation sequence of RBCs; nuclear chromatin is clumped yielding a round nucleus in dark-blue cytoplasm; nucleoli are present but may not always be visible

Prostacyclin: Substance produced by the endothelium and capable of dilating vessels and inhibiting platelet aggregation

Protamine sulfate test: Measure of the presence of soluble fibrin monomers

Protein C: Serine proteases that acts in concert with protein S to inhibit coagulation cofactors and inactivate inhibitors of plasminogen activators

Protein S: Hemostasis cofactor that acts in concert with protein C

Prothrombin: Inactive precursor to thrombin

Prothrombin family: Coagulation factors II, VII, IX, and X

Prothrombin time: Screening test for abnormalities in the extrinsic coagulation pathway and for monitoring coumarin therapy

Prussian blue stain: Special stain used to identify non-heme iron

PT: Prothrombin time

Purpura: General term for bleeding from capillaries into the skin and mucosa

Pyknosis: Cells with extremely condensed nuclear chromatin characteristic of cellular degeneration

Pyropoikilocytosis: RBCs with extreme variation in cell shape caused by sensitivity to heat

Pyruvate kinase: Enzyme in the Embden-Meyerhof glycolytic pathway; a deficiency of the enzyme creates a congenital non-spherocytic hemolytic anemia

RBC: Red blood cell

RDW: Red cell distribution width

Red blood cell indices: See mean cell volume, mean cell hemoglobin, and mean cell hemoglobin concentration

Red cell distribution width (RDW): Coefficient of variation of RBC volume

Red marrow: Site within the bone marrow that produces blood cells

Reider cleft: Split or indentation in the lymphocyte nucleus causing the nucleus to resemble the buttocks

Reticulocyte: Precursor cell in the maturation sequence of RBCs; no nucleus is present and the cytoplasm is bluish-pink; RNA in the cell precipitates with supravital staining

Reticulocytosis: Absolute reticulocyte count above 108×10^9/liter

Ristocetin: Reagent used in platelet aggregation studies

Rouleaux: RBCs appearing as stacks of coins

Rubriblast: Earliest recognizable cell of the erythrocytic series

Rubricyte: Intermediate precursor in the maturation sequence of RBCs; the nucleus has a checkered appearance with areas of densely clumped chromatin; the cytoplasm is gray

Russell body: Globules of gamma globulins in the cytoplasm of plasma cells

Satellitism: Platelets adhering to the periphery of neutrophils as a result of contact with EDTA; artifactual

Schilling test: Measure of vitamin B_{12} absorption by the gastrointestinal tract

Schistocyte: See schizocyte

Schizocyte: Schistocyte; fragmented RBC

Scurvy: Deficiency of vitamin C leading to an acquired abnormality of the basement membrane of blood vessels; other systemic abnormalities also are seen

Sea-blue histiocytosis: Autosomal recessive disorder causing an enzyme deficiency; resultant failure to break down lipids results in large macrophages with blue-green cytoplasm

Secondary fibrinolysis: Hemostatic disorder caused by excess clot formation which leads to consumption of coagulation factors and platelets, as well as increased clot degradation

Segmented neutrophil: Mature granulocyte; it is distinguished from the earlier cell by the segmented nucleus with lobes attached by filaments

Senile purpura: Bleeding into the tissue due to atrophy of subcutaneous tissue

Serine protease: Enzymes that have serine as the active site

Shift to the left: Increase in the number of immature WBCs in the peripheral blood

Sickle cell: See drepanocyte

Sickle cell anemia: Hemolytic disorder resulting from the homozygous inheritance of genes that produce abnormal beta chains in hemoglobin; the hemoglobin is less soluble than normal hemoglobin under reduced oxygen conditions leading to RBCs that are irreversibly sickled

Sickle cell trait: Heterozygous inheritance of a gene that produces abnormal beta chains in hemoglobin; since one normal gene also is inherited, some normal beta chains are produced and hemolysis may not be evident unless extreme oxygen deprivation occurs

Sideroblast: NRBC with deposits of free iron in the cytoplasm

Sideroblastic anemia: Disorder in which the body adequately stores iron but the iron cannot be utilized

Siderocyte: Non-nucleated RBC with deposits of free iron in the cytoplasm

Siderotic granules: RBC cytoplasmic inclusions appearing as a small blue specks and consisting of non-heme iron; siderotic granules usually occur in clusters near the periphery of the RBC; their presence may be confirmed with a Prussian blue stain

Smudge cell: Artifacts due to mechanical trauma of blood smear preparation; the nucleus is distorted and separated from the cytoplasm

Sodium citrate: Anticoagulant commonly used for collection of specimens for coagulation studies; it acts as a calcium chelator, thus deleting a vital component of the coagulation mechanism

Spherocyte: Ball-shaped RBC with no central pallor

Sphingomyelinase: Enzyme that may be deficient in patients with Niemann-Pick disease

Splenomegaly: Enlargement of the spleen

Staphylokinase: Therapeutic agent derived from staphylococci and used to initiate fibrinolysis

Stem cell: Blood cell precursor

Sterile gut syndrome: Bleeding episodes following antibiotic therapy that has eliminated normal, vitamin K–producing, intestinal flora; without vitamin K, non-functional coagulation factors are produced

Stomatocyte: Round RBC with an elongated, mouth-like area of central pallor

Storage pool disease: Inheritance of one of a group of disorders having platelet granules with abnormal release response

Streptokinase: Therapeutic agent derived from beta-hemolytic streptococci and used to initiate fibrinolysis

Stuart-Prower factor: Coagulation factor X; inactive precursor to a serine protease in the intrinsic coagulation pathway

Stypven time: Coagulation test used to differentiate between deficiencies of factors VII or X

Substitution studies: Tests in which patient plasma is mixed with normal plasma, aged serum, or adsorbed plasma; aid in identifying factor deficiencies

Substrate: Substance upon which an enzyme acts

Sucrose hemolysis test: See sugar water test

Sugar water test: Measure of RBC sensitivity to complement attachment; positive tests usually are associated with paroxysmal nocturnal hemoglobinuria

Sulfhemoglobin: Hemoglobin molecule that has irreversibly reacted with sulfur compounds

Supravital stain: Stain in which the cells react with a dye while they are living

Target cell: See codocyte

Tay-Sachs disease: Autosomal recessive disorder causing a deficiency of hexosaminidase; the failure to break down lipids results in vacuolated lymphocytes and histiocytes, as well as other systemic abnormalities

TdT: Terminal deoxynucleotidyl transferase

Teardrop cell: See dacryocyte

Telangiectasia: Spider-like dilations of small vessels

Terminal deoxynucleotidyl transferase (TdT): Cell marker useful in identifying early lymphocytes

Thalassemia: Hemoglobin disorder in which insufficient quantities of one of the globin chains are produced; the deficiency leads to a microcytic, hypochromic anemia; classification is designated by the deficient globin chain

Thorn cell: See acanthocyte

Thrombin: Enzyme that splits fibrinogen, stimulates platelet aggregation, and activates cofactors and protein C

Thrombin time: Measure of quantitative and qualitative defects of fibrinogen

Thrombocyte: Platelet

Thrombocytopathy: Functional disorder of platelets

Thrombocytopenia: Absolute platelet count below 140×10^9/liter

Thrombocytosis: Absolute platelet count above 415×10^9/liter

Thrombogenic: Capable of forming blood clots

Thrombomodulin: Substance produced by the endothelium and capable of neutralizing thrombin and enhancing the activity of protein C

Thromboplastin: Tissue factor that activates factor VII in the coagulation mechanism

Thrombopoiesis: Production of platelets

Thrombopoietin: Substance that regulates the proliferation of platelets

Thrombotic: Capable of producing clots

Thrombotic thrombocytopenic purpura: Intravascular platelet aggregation possibly caused by decreased prostacyclin production

Thromboxane: Aggregating agent and vaso-constrictor

TIBC: Total iron binding capacity

Tissue basophil: Tissue cell that plays a role in allergic reactions

Tissue eosinophil: Fixed tissue variant of the motile eosinophil

Tissue neutrophil: Fixed tissue cells with neutrophilic granules

Tissue plasminogen activator: Serine protease produced by the endothelium and capable of activating the fibrinolytic system

T lymphocyte: WBC that undergoes differentiation in the thymus and is responsible for cellular immunity

Tourniquet test: Measure of capillary fragility

Toxic granulation: Small, dark-staining granules within the cytoplasm of neutrophils; often associated with bacterial infections

Transaminase: Enzyme that creates covalent bonds in the unstable clot resulting in a stable clot

Transferrin: Glycoprotein that transports iron

Triangle cell: See knizocyte

Urea solubility test: Measure of the presence of factor XIII

Urobilinogen: Compound formed when bilirubin is degraded

Urokinase: Proteolytic enzyme that is found in body fluids and activates fibrinolysis

Variant lymphocyte: Lymphocyte that has been stimulated by an antigen; also known as reactive, stimulated, and atypical

Vein: Blood vessel that carries deoxygenated blood from tissues to the heart

von Willebrand's disease: Inherited bleeding disorder caused by a deficiency of von Willebrand's factor

von Willebrand's factor: High-molecular-weight substance produced by the endothelium and capable of binding to the subendothelium and supporting platelet adhesion

Waldenström's macroglobulinemia: Lymphocytic malignancy resulting in overproduction of IgM

WBC: White blood cell

Whole blood clot lysis: Measure of clot degradation

Wright's stain: Romanosky stain; polychrome stain useful in WBC differentiation, as well as RBC and platelet morphologic evaluation

Xerocytosis: Hereditary RBC defect that allows water to exit the RBC; characterized by codocytes and RBCs with hemoglobin concentrated in one area of the cell

Yellow marrow: Site within the bone marrow composed of fat and not producing blood cells

Zymogen: Enzyme precursor

Index

Note: Page numbers followed by f indicate figures.